Heidi Moretti, MS, RD

gut
fix

Discover the Herbal Remedies,
Diet Tips, _and_ Supplements
Clinically Shown to Heal Your Gut

First published by The Healthy RD 2023

This book is informational only and is not intended as a substitute for medical advice from your healthcare provider. You should consult a healthcare provider, such as a qualified medical doctor, on matters relating to your health and particularly regarding any symptoms that require medical attention.

First edition

ISBN: 979-8-9884698-0-3

Editing by Sandy Draper

This book was professionally typeset on Reedsy.
Find out more at reedsy.com

This book is dedicated to you, my wonderful readers, who are brave enough to go beyond the status quo and take your own path to health.

"Your gut is not Las Vegas. What happens in the gut does not stay in the gut."

Peter Kozlowski, MD, Unfunc Your Gut

Contents

Preface

The Guts of the Issue

If you picked up this book thinking you are one of the unlucky few afflicted with gut health issues, let me assure you that you are not alone. In fact, worldwide, 40 percent of people suffer from at least one digestive disease. In comparison, around 66 percent of people in the US struggle with one or more **digestive diseases**,[1] including gastroesophageal reflux disease, gallbladder disease, inflammatory bowel diseases, and others. More money is spent on digestive remedies than heart or mental health, too, at over $136 billion per year. So why, in our so-called progressive society, are digestive issues so prevalent, and how do you find relief?

As a clinician and researcher with twenty-four years of experience, I'm passionate about gut health. This is because it is at the root of most ailments, and because of this, achieving gut health is the quickest path to feeling vitality again. Because I'm also trained in functional medicine, I have learned many techniques to help get people on the path to feeling well. In my experience, patients feel better quickly and usually permanently using this functional medicine approach. When, in fact, they previously only found temporary or no relief after trying conventional interactions with their gastrointestinal doctor.

To be clear, traditional medicine does have its place, and I urge you to visit your provider if you're having gut issues to get a complete diagnosis. Still, it is worth knowing that there is more to treating your gut issue than conventional medicine. What's more, if you're having gut trouble, but your doctor can't find the problem using a scope, scan, or other tests, you may be told there is nothing wrong with you and given little or no advice on how to feel better. And if you do receive a diagnosis of, for example, Crohn's disease or Irritable Bowel Syndrome (IBS), you may find that the medication for your specific gut disorder only masks the issue rather than treating the root cause.

Getting to the Root Cause

As you will discover in this book, the root cause of many gut issues is a lack of essential nutrients and building blocks for the gut. For example, a lack of sufficient nutrients causes gut cells to be inflamed, function poorly, cause pain and discomfort, or all of the above. Additionally, lacking the nutritional building blocks due to stressful situations or an imbalanced diet can disrupt your body's ability to digest foods well. This can be a root cause of distress in your gut and throughout your whole body.

Genetics may play a partial role in these gut conditions, but your genes don't tell the whole story. Genes may load the gun, so to speak, but diet and lifestyle pull the trigger on these diseases. There is an entire field dedicated to how food and nutrients control how our genes express themselves called epigenetics.[2] Epigenetics, in simple terms, is the effect of your food and your environment on how well your genes work. In other words, what you eat has a huge impact on whether your genes cause damage to your body or not. This is good news for all of us because we can make simple diet and lifestyle changes to reduce gut symptoms even due to daunting genetic conditions. And understanding that food significantly impacts your health's destiny is much more potent than feeling helpless due to genes.

Yet, many medical doctors ignore the basic building blocks of the gut: food, herbs, healing compounds, and nutrients. This is largely because medical doctors aren't taught these critical healing tools in their academic training. In my experience, my patients feel better so much more quickly from a nutritional approach than any other mode of treatment for digestive issues in most cases. I'll be sharing some of their stories in this book. And I think you'll find that if you are willing to try some targeted nutritional support supplements and improve your diet, you will create your own personalized gut fix and discover the healing solution you've been searching for.

Using This Book

Knowledge is power, so we'll journey through the digestive tract and where and how issues might develop.

So, if you're ready, let's dive into the ultimate gut fix, knowledge, and finding the right nutritional balance.

[1] Almario C, Ballal M, et al. Burden of gastrointestinal symptoms in the United States: results of a nationally representative survey of over 71,000 Americans. *Am J Gastroenterol.* 2018 Nov;113(11):1701–10.

[2] Lorenzo P, Izquierdo A, et al. Epigenetic effects of healthy foods and lifestyle habits from the Southern European Atlantic diet pattern: A narrative review. *Adv Nutr.* 2022 Oct 2;13(5):1725–47.

1

Chapter 1

Digestion 101: The Inner Workings of the Digestive System

In this chapter, you will learn about the basics of gut structure and health through a nutritional lens and why gut ailments are so common.

Figure 1: The flow of food through the digestive tract starts in the oral cavity (mouth) and then moves down to the anus. Important organs for the digestive tract include the liver, gallbladder, and pancreas.

Salivary glands ——————— Oral cavity

Pharynx ——————

Oesophagus

Liver ——————

Gall bladder ——————

Pancreas ——————
Small intestine ——————
Large intestine ——————

Rectum ——————
Anus ——————

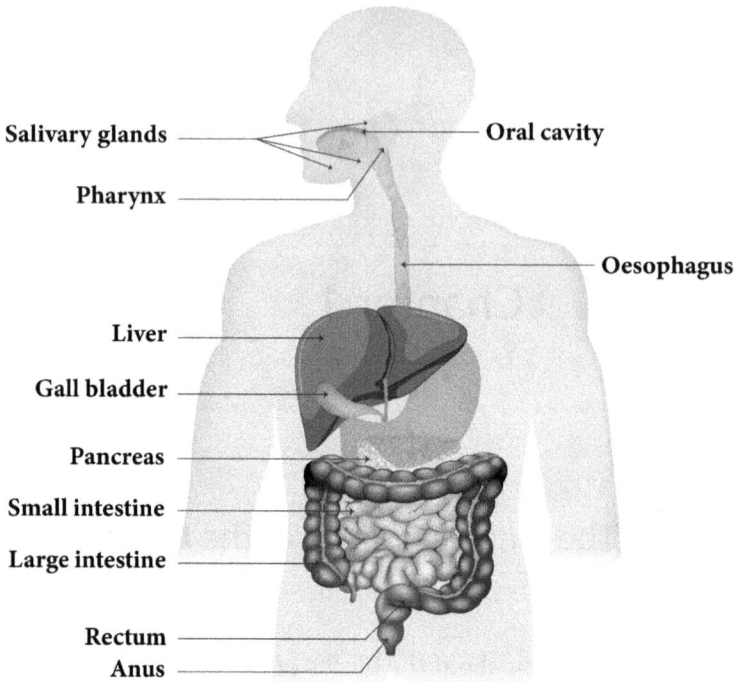

How Digestion Begins

The second you smell the aroma of food, your body starts anticipating eating. That mouth-watering effect primes your digestive tract for what comes next—your first bite of food. Digestive enzymes and saliva secrete into your mouth to lubricate each mouthful and start to break down each morsel as you munch and chew.

Your whole gut, including your mouth, has healthy bacteria and other microbes, known as a **microbiome**, that control a lot of your body's functioning. But your mouth needs help to produce these digestive enzymes. In times gone by, foods were rich in natural enzymes and healthy bacteria, but in the modern world of packaged foods, they are often killed by heat processing and refining long before they reach your dinner plate.

Chewing your food helps to mechanically break it down into smaller pieces. But today's commonly eaten foods are so soft that even the chewing process is altered. Foods like donuts, burgers, pizza, cereal, French fries, chips, and other processed foods require minimal chewing. The result is that the food spends less time in your mouth getting broken down. This hurries the food into your stomach, cutting the digestive process short. Combine this with the fact that many Westernized foods are basically void of many nutrients and healthy compounds, and digestion doesn't get off to the best start. In addition, chemical fertilizers, additives, and preservatives contain highly sensitive compounds which can disrupt the gut lining.

Contrast our modern diet to our ancestors who dined out on hard-to-chew meats on the bone, fish, and organ meats that are a bit tough in texture but extremely rich in nutrients, fibrous vegetables, roots, herbs, seeds, honey, and the like. These foods mostly require a lot of chewing. These unprocessed foods are naturally rich in enzymes that promote digestive function and are rich in natural **antioxidants** and probiotics, as well as nutrients for the whole body and gut. Our ancestral diet slowed down the first part of the digestive process, making it easier to digest foods. Sadly, these foods today, even if available, often lack nutrients, and we will get into more of the causes of this in Chapter 2.

The traditional use of herbs combined with these simple ancestral foods had unique benefits to help the digestive processes. Containing antioxidants and healing compounds, these herbs often soothed and coated the gut's digestive lining while destroying unwanted germs and bacteria.

Stomach and Esophageal Health

As we swallow food into the esophagus, its muscles move the food particles along the way. From the esophagus, food enters the stomach, where some major digestive processes occur primarily due to the acidity of the stomach and enzyme production. This acid helps activate enzymes, break down protein, and keep food propelling through the digestive tract.

Did You Know . . . Genetics Is Not Necessarily to Blame

Esophageal cancer cases are rising due to increased gastric or acid reflux, ironically related to a poor diet. There is also an increase in inflammatory conditions related to food intolerances, i.e., eosinophilic esophagitis. This condition was rare, but now at least two in a hundred people undergoing endoscopy for any reason have it.[1] Our genes haven't changed much. What has changed is our food supply. Eosinophilic esophagitis is thought to be predominantly a food-related allergic condition rooted in gut imbalances. We will get into more of why there are more problems with acid reflux and esophageal issues throughout the text.

A majorly essential but underappreciated part of the stomach and digestive tract is the mucus lining, which helps create around 10 liters of mucus per day. That's 40 cups of mucus per day! It is a gel-like substance that helps carry away unwanted and harmful compounds while protecting the stomach and intestinal cells from damage. In your gut, you have a mucus layer attached to the intestine and another unattached layer with more liquid. Mucus production is affected by what you eat, and many herbs can help your body increase its protective mucus production.

Figure 2: The gut lining produces 40 cups of protective mucus daily in a healthy gut. This crucial lining protects the body from harmful germs and toxins and helps prevent inflammatory reactions.

---

[1] Dellon E, Hirano I. Epidemiology and natural history of eosinophilic esophagitis. *Gastroenterology.* 2018 Jan;154(2):319–32.e3.

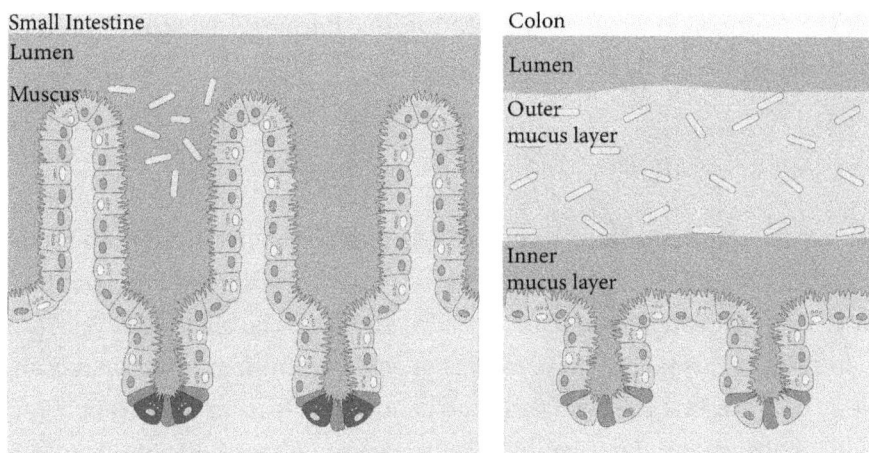

When there is a disruption in the integrity of the mucus lining, the gut is susceptible to bacteria, **inflammation**, and more. Some scientists believe that damage to this lining is one of the major causes of severe digestive diseases like ulcerative colitis and that strengthening mucus production through diet and nutrition may be highly beneficial.[2, 3] In Chapter 4, I have included an extensive section on how to help treat stomach issues with a natural approach when possible.

Did You Know . . . Acid Reflux Has Little to Do with Acidity

Acid reflux isn't necessarily related to acid at all. Still, it remains a significant problem in the United States, with up to 25 percent of people struggling with gastroesophageal reflux disease (**GERD**). Even more disturbing is that the rates of GERD continue to worsen among young people. Between 50 to 80

---

[2] Johansson M, Sjövall H, et al. The gastrointestinal mucus system in health and disease. *Nat Rev Gastroenterol Hepatol.* 2013 Jun;10(6):352–61.

[3] Paone P, Cani P. Mucus barrier, mucins and gut microbiota: The expected slimy partners? *Gut.* 2020;69: 2232–43.

percent of the population suffer from symptoms like fullness, heartburn, nausea, anorexia, regurgitation, bloating, and burping.[4] The collective term for these symptoms is functional dyspepsia.

The Small Intestine and Biliary Tree

The most complicated and orchestrated digestive events occur in the small intestine because most of your food's nutrients are absorbed into your body here. Your gallbladder and pancreas, also known as the biliary tree, perform their roles at this point. Here, a bolus of acid-neutralizing compounds and many enzymes are released from the pancreas to further break down your food for absorption. Your gallbladder releases a large volume of bile to help you digest and absorb fats and fat-soluble vitamins.

The lining of the small intestine continuously produces most of your digestive enzymes. Within that lining, as you may recall from earlier, is mucus that adheres to the intestinal wall and protects it from germs and damaging chemicals. Ideally, any toxins get passed along into the large intestine and out of the body. But today's diets undoubtedly cause disruption in this mucus lining and the enzymes you need to break down food, causing inflammation and more. This makes us susceptible to many of the common gut ailments we have today.

One of the most challenging aspects of the small intestine, however, is that it isn't reachable with scopes, so identifying and treating conditions is next to impossible. However, there are increasing ways to rule out issues such as small intestinal bacterial overgrowth (SIBO), which continues to be a more common issue than once thought.

It is also hard to identify issues with the biliary tree until it is too late. Processed foods and poor eating patterns contribute to our ever-increasing gallbladder problems. Additionally, there can be sludge and inflammation

---

[4] Sperber A, Bangdiwala S, et al. Worldwide prevalence and burden of functional gastrointestinal disorders, results of Rome foundation global study. *Gastroenterology.* 2021 Jan;160(1):99–114.e3.

from poor diets in the biliary tree, reducing the pancreas's release of enzymes. This further worsens inflammation and damage in the small intestine due to poorly absorbed food compounds.

As a result of all this **inflammation** and poorly absorbed food along with highly reactive foods, an increased intestinal permeability can occur. This is often called leaky gut. Leaky gut causes unwanted and poorly digested compounds to enter the bloodstream. These compounds directly affect the body's immune response, sending out threat signals throughout the body. The body thinks it is being attacked by foreign invaders, and the immune system goes into overdrive to fight response. Due to your body's **fight-or-flight response**, inflammation occurs at a magnified level throughout the body and even the brain.

As you can see, problems starting in the mouth related to food quality can create a snowball effect of problems further down the digestive tract.

Did You Know . . . Signs of a Leaky Gut

Symptoms of a leaky gut can appear anywhere in the body, including the skin, hair, joints, heart, muscles, and more. For many people, including me, the most obvious sign of a leaky gut is skin inflammation, including cystic acne, eczema, psoriasis, and more. Eliminating food sensitivities often gives the gut a chance to heal. One of the first pleasant signs of gut healing is a reduction in unsightly skin issues and digestive complaints.

The Large Intestine and Its Microbiome

The body absorbs fluids and electrolyte minerals from your diet in the large intestine. Probiotic bacteria live in the large intestine; they ferment fiber and feed on the probiotics from your diet. This is also where some of the primary fuel for the gut is made, called **short-chain fatty acids**. This fuel is made from the fermentation process of undigested whole foods. These bacteria also do some fascinating work in helping you digest and absorb vitamins and minerals. Many healthy gut bacteria have enzymes that further break down foods for improved digestion of nutrients.

Not surprisingly, your gut bacteria, also known as the **microbiome**, vary vastly, and some experts believe that your gut probiotics are as unique to you as your fingerprint.[5] Sadly, a typical Western diet can disrupt the balance of the microbiome, causing lots of intestinal distress. Sugars (i.e., refined carbohydrates such as pastries, white bread and pasta, and candy) can severely disrupt the microbiome balance, for example. But you can do plenty to support your gut health and bring it into balance, and we'll be exploring those remedies in later chapters.

Did You Know . . . A Disrupted Microbiome Can Lead to Ill-Health

Long-term or extensive microbiome disruption is linked to increased mood disorders such as depression and anxiety. It is even linked to heart disease, Alzheimer's, autoimmune diseases, cancer, liver disease, skin disorders, and more.[6] All told, the microbiome is responsible for a considerable amount of your overall health, so finding a balance in your gut is critical to your health.

---

[5] Cryan J, O'Mahony S. The microbiome-gut-brain axis: from bowel to behavior. *Neurogastroenterol Motil.* 2011 Mar;23(3):187–92.

[6] Vijay A, Valdes A. Role of the gut microbiome in chronic diseases: A narrative review. *Eur J Clin Nutr.* 2022 Apr;76(4):489–501.

2

Chapter 2

Why Diet Just Isn't Enough

You've probably heard it many times, "supplements are a waste of time" or "stop taking supplements" from either news sources or ill-informed doctors. Not surprisingly, most doctors today are "deficient" in diet knowledge due to receiving little to no training in nutrition in medical school. According to the Association of American Medical Colleges, only 20 percent of medical schools provide any nutrition training, and most doctors average less than twenty hours of total nutrition training in their whole career.[7] This is even true of gastrointestinal doctors, which is somewhat mind-boggling given the exclusive role of the gut in absorbing food and nutrients. In contrast, dietitians receive around twenty hours of nutrition education each week of undergrad training and more in graduate school. For nutritionists like me, nutrition training is over 4,200 hours before graduating with a master's degree. And personally, I haven't stopped learning about nutrients since

---

[7] School of Medicine. Why medical schools need to focus more on nutrition. *School of Medicine.* https://med.stanford.edu/school/leadership/dean/precision-health-in-the-news/why-me dica-schools-need-focus-nutrition.html.

then.

Granted, there are exceptions, as some doctors have a profound desire to heal, so they self-teach nutrition. And some dietitians also care very little about the healing process and are highly influenced by the power of Big Food and Big Pharma. Generally, however, nutrition advice in the world is often lacking critical thinking and leads many people astray, especially when it comes to supplements. As a nutrition practitioner for over twenty years, I have conducted and published clinical research on vitamins, so I can say with authority that negative headlines about supplements are not doing anyone any good. And the comments and headlines telling you to avoid supplements are flat-out misguided for most people. They are also way too generic to suit you as a unique individual.

Since you are reading this book, you likely realize that anti-supplement media hype is untrue and probably had some success feeling better when taking various dietary supplements. You should be proud of yourself for taking positive steps toward improving your health.

Why Supplement?

The only supplements that likely cause any significant level of harm are usually bodybuilding "natural" steroids or stimulants, as these pose health risks. But there are countless reasons why certain dietary supplements can help you. They range from spices and herbs to whole food compounds and antioxidants, as well as vitamins and minerals. Not only are they vastly different from each other, but some can literally be life-changing when chosen well.

Regarding gut health, there are some truly healing supplements on the market, and by reading this book, you'll discover when and how to use them best. There are some valid reasons and scenarios when you might want to avoid certain supplements, but they are fewer than you might realize. While the benefits of taking dietary supplements usually far exceed the reasons not to, it is all about making informed decisions. However, you should always review any new supplements with a healthcare provider well-versed in nutrition to ensure they are a good choice for you.

There are six main reasons to include dietary supplements if you struggle with gut issues or are just trying to be healthier. First, modern food production methods mean our food is becoming less and less nutritious— even if you eat whole foods. Second, ancestral ways of eating (the diet our bodies are designed to eat) have been abandoned. Next, the chemicals in food alter gut health, whether listed on the label or not. It is also tough to resist and avoid processed foods, alcohol, and sugar because they are everywhere, and these foods deplete nutrients and antioxidants. Around half of Americans are also on prescription medications that deplete nutrients. Last, gut cells can repair quickly if you give them what you need. We will explore all of these reasons in more depth next.

Foods Today Are Lacking

Let's face it: a carrot in today's grocery store is not the same carrot that was grown by your great-grandparents. Today, the soil is inundated with chemical fertilizers that encourage growth but leave food lacking in its naturally abundant nutrient and antioxidant qualities. This is because chemical fertilizers are simply nitrogen, phosphorus, and potassium. But there is much more to growing food that affects the nutrient content of foods.

In traditional farming methods, the only fertilizers were natural compost made from manure and decomposing plants. These complex soil compounds make humus, which is rich in probiotics, trace minerals, and nutrients. Humus makes each piece of food grown on them more able to absorb nutrients from the soil and, frankly, taste much better.

Sadly, the longer crops are grown with synthetic fertilizers, the less nutritious they become, and your body suffers. This means you are likely low in the essential vitamins and minerals required for proper gut function.

While some farmers and ranchers are returning to regenerative agriculture practices, there is a long way to go to get our soil rich again. But **regenerative farming** increases the vitamins, minerals, and antioxidants of your food, so you should always try to choose foods grown regenerative if you can. But until there is an agricultural revolution, you will thrive better with more nutrients and antioxidants from supplementation, and this has been borne out countless times in my practice and in my own life.

Ancestral Foods Have Gone by the Wayside

Remember the low-fat craze? It is now sneakily being replaced by the latest trends and scare tactics to lure us into buying similarly gimmicky packaged foods. Before dietary guidelines, people ate whole foods, natural foods, period. Current diet crazes and dogmatic eating practices cause us to be too restrictive with our diets. For example, people are replacing whole foods like homemade bone broth chicken soup with boneless, skinless chicken breasts and fat-free chicken bouillon instead, which is stripped of many of its nutrients. The introduction of fake meats is also questionable as they are highly processed. Sadly, we rarely return from the processed propaganda put before us as a society.

We were meant to eat more holistically than that. For example, chicken liver and organ meats are the most nutritious parts of the chicken and shouldn't be tossed out. They provide vital nutrients. Vegetarians used to eat more holistically as well. Unlike our ancestors, our food often travels long distances and loses a lot of its nutrients by the time it gets to our plates. In other words, we need to return to holistic eating by using real food. But supplements are often required because our foods are so far removed from whole.

Chemicals in Foods Alter Your Gut

Whether you know it or not, your food contains many chemicals, even if the packaging claims it is "all-natural." An excellent example of this is whole wheat products. Farmers, under pressure to provide high yields, use **desiccation**. This means right before harvesting the crop, they spray glyphosate (Roundup®) on wheat or other grains to quickly and uniformly ripen them. This chemical cannot be rinsed or cooked off, so we end up eating it. I find that even health food stores struggle to keep foods free of products with chemicals. In addition, there are over 10,000 chemicals in our food supply that have questionable safety for gut health and the whole body.[8],[9] Strikingly, around 99 percent of these chemicals were approved by Big Industry and have never been evaluated by the FDA, according to the Environmental Working Group.[10] Ultimately, this means we need more probiotics and healing compounds than ever, and supplementing can be helpful.

Did You Know . . . It Is Wise to Be Wary of Glyphosate

Glyphosate disrupts the bacteria in your gut and may contribute to a host of health issues, including many digestive disorders. Unless you choose USDA organic foods, your foods contain many chemicals. If you eat in a restaurant or don't specifically know where your foods come from, the odds are they contain gut-stripping chemicals.

Hard to Resist Processed Foods

Most of us try to eat as best as possible, but human nature makes it almost impossible to resist processed foods altogether. This is because we are hard-wired to eat more food and especially more highly palatable foods like these. Our bodies are wise to do so because, for most of the time humans have been on the planet, we have faced starvation more than we have abundance. Our hormones and biological drives tell us to eat, eat, eat.

---

[8] Tracy B. FDA hasn't reviewed some food additives in decades. CBS News, CBS Interactive. 2023 Feb 22. https://www.cbsnews.com/news/fda-food-additives-safety-review-california -legislation/

[9] U.S. Food & Drug Administration. Food additive status list. FDA. https://www.fda.gov/food/ food-additives-petitions/food-additive-status-list

[10] Benesh M. EWG analysis: Almost all new food chemicals greenlighted by industry, not the FDA. EWG. 2022 Apr 13. https://www.ewg.org/news-insights/news/2022/04/ewg-analysis- almost-all-new-food-chemicals-greenlighted-industry-not-fda

So, it's not your fault when you indulge in junk food. We all do it. Despite our best efforts, we almost all cave into cravings sometimes, and the food manufacturers know this. These ultra-processed foods are not only devoid of most nutrients that help heal and repair the gut, but they also rob the body of nutrients and antioxidants because of their high **free-radical** content.

And I'm talking about all processed foods, organic or not. After all, organic pizza is still made with highly processed grains with little to no nutritional value. Historically, your body, especially your gut, is ill-equipped to handle all these processed foods. And many of these modern foods lack nutrients, so no wonder the US population is getting more significant health issues; they are exposed to many nutrient-robbing foods. This makes micronutrient requirements higher than the outdated **RDI** amounts for most people.

All told, this just means that we need supplements in our diets to compensate for the processed foods in front of us.

Prescription Medications Rob You of Nutrients

According to the National Center for Health Statistics, around 65 percent of Americans take at least one prescription drug.[11] Most medications, including for cholesterol and blood pressure, deplete multiple nutrients. These nutrients are required for proper gut function, meaning that a massive part of the population is in a nutrient deficit that they will never crawl out of unless they take the appropriate supplements.

Give Gut Cells What They Need

While these scary statistics might make you think it is impossible to have a healthy gut, it also has tremendous healing abilities. This is because digestive cells reproduce every five days, and so if you make improvements in your diet and feed your gut healing compounds through diet and supplements, most

---

[11] Centers for Disease Control and Prevention. Products - Data Briefs - Number 347 - August 2019. CDC. 2019 Aug 14. https://www.cdc.gov/nchs/products/databriefs/db347.htm.

often, you can and will feel better quickly. I've seen this happen many times in my practice. But you need to move away from the mindset that your foods will give you enough to heal because they are often deficient in nutrients.

3

Chapter 3

What's Lacking in a Gut-Healthy Diet

Did you know that the gut lining is only one cell thick? When you understand this, you can also understand how vulnerable it is to changes in your diet. Each cell in your body requires nutrients as building blocks for proper structure and function. But I have yet to meet anyone who gets enough nourishment in their diet alone. I know this by doing countless food recalls over my 20-plus-year career as a dietitian. I also know this because research shows that people can be low in any nutrient and that each individual falls short in at least one, but likely more, nutrients.[12]

As I described at the end of the previous chapter, the good news is that the gut lining can rebuild in about five days. So, when you improve your nutrient intake, you also enhance the strength and resilience of your gut lining.

You may be wondering just how a lack of nutrients causes gut issues. The true answer is in countless ways, and this chapter could be a whole book in and of itself. But, I will try to summarize as best as possible so you get the idea of how a lack of nutrients causes a broad array of gut issues.

_____

[12] Kumar M, Pal N, et al. Omega-3 fatty acids and their interaction with the gut microbiome in the prevention and amelioration of type-2 diabetes. *Nutrients.* 2022 Apr 21;14(9):1723.

Protector of Gut Health—Omega-3

Omega-3 fatty acids are an essential type of fat integral to the structure of cell walls and cellular signaling related to immunity and more. New research even shows omega-3s help regulate the number and diversity of healthy bacteria in the gut. [13] [14] Eating healthy omega-3 fats also helps protect gut cells from damaging inflammatory compounds.

And without a doubt, this is a nutrient that most of us fall short of. This is because we should eat fresh fish regularly. But you need to eat about 3 oz of salmon daily to get the ideal amount for your gut health. This equals the number of grams of omega-3 in a single cod liver or fish oil supplement. As you can see, you need more omega-3 fats for health than your diet alone can provide.

Sadly, the American public has been convinced that plant sources of omega-3 are equal to oily fish omega-3 fats. Unfortunately, it just isn't true. Plant-derived omega-3s have the potential to become active in the body, but as it turns out, only about 3 percent at most becomes active. Our genes also regulate this process, so some people do not effectively convert any plant sources into activated omega-3 in the body.

Protein: The Building Blocks of Gut Health

Protein is one of the primary building blocks of cells, including your intestinal cells. Even gut probiotics are made of protein. So, as you can imagine, protein plays an integral role in gut health. Too little protein in the diet significantly increases frailty as we age. If you live in the United States, you will think that

---

[13] Corsetti G, Romano C, et al. Qualitative nitrogen malnutrition damages gut and alters microbiome in adult mice. A preliminary histopathological study. *Nutrients.* 2021 Mar 26;13(4):1089.

[14] Barekatain R, Chrystal P, et al. Performance, intestinal permeability, and gene expression of selected tight junction proteins in broiler chickens fed reduced protein diets supplemented with arginine, glutamine, and glycine subjected to a leaky gut model. *Poult Sci.* 2019 Dec 1;98(12):6761–71.

protein malnutrition couldn't exist. It does, even in young adults. I often see this scenario, especially in my vegan and vegetarian patients. The source, concentration, and your whole body's protein needs significantly contribute to your gut health. Fascinatingly, early research shows that low protein diets, as would be in the case of many restrictive diets today, causes the gut lining to become leaky (see also Chapter 1, page 8). [15] This allows bacteria to spread to the liver, the spleen, and other organs, creating inflammation throughout the body and brain.

Popular culture has led us to believe beans and legumes are good protein sources. But, to equal 3 oz of salmon, you would have to eat 1.5 cups of black beans, while vegans and vegetarians would have to eat this amount multiple times daily to meet their protein needs. Can you or anyone imagine eating 5 cups of beans a day? Or eating the equivalent amount of soy or tofu? And even if you do, the protein isn't adequate in quality due to many other factors, as you will soon learn.

That's not to say that certain kinds of beans and soy can't be a source of protein as well as fiber and nutrients in the diet, but the omnivore's gut doesn't adapt well to eating them in the massive amounts required to get enough protein. Let's find out why.

Not long ago, the world thought the only way to keep your microbiome healthy was to eat fiber and probiotics. While these factors remain helpful, protein intake and quality play a significant role in the amount and diversity of your microbiome. For example, when animals are undernourished in protein, they have a decrease in healthy bacteria amounts, including *Lactobacillus bacteria.* When given high-quality protein, the numbers and ratios of beneficial bacteria increase.

Other studies show that the ratios of gut bacteria are improved if animals are given milk protein, fish protein, or other animal protein instead of soy

---

[15] Zhu Y, Lin X, et al. Meat, dairy and plant proteins alter bacterial composition of rat gut bacteria. *Sci Rep.* 2015;5:15220.

protein.[16] Researchers showed that the amino acid balance and digestibility of dietary protein are primary factors that contribute to the composition, structure, and function of gut microbes in humans.[17] In addition, the **antinutritional components** of plant proteins limit their digestive ability, and researchers speculate this could be why they can negatively affect the microbiome.[18] [19] [20]

Beneficial compounds made in the gut called **postbiotics** also increase with a higher protein in the diet. For example, more short-chain fatty acids are produced when you eat an adequate amount of protein. By comparison, too much protein or protein from questionable animal sources may also disrupt the gut, so finding the right balance is critical. Keeping your protein intake at around 1 g/kg per day, or 0.43g per pound of body weight, is now considered ideal, contrary to the **RDI**.[21] So, if you weigh 170 lbs, the protein you would need daily is about 73 g, or between 7−8 oz of high-quality protein per day.

Fueling Gut Health with Collagen

Collagen is essentially connective tissue, so it comes from many protein-rich foods. It is found in bone broth, gelatin, chicken skin, fish skin and bones, organ meats, cartilage, and slow-cooked bone-in meats.

---

[16] Wu S, Bhat Z, et al. Effect of dietary protein and processing on gut microbiota—a systematic review. *Nutrients.* 2022;14: 453.

[17] Farsijani S, Cauley J, et al. Relation between dietary protein intake and gut microbiome composition in community-dwelling older men: Findings from the osteoporotic fractures in men study (MrOS). *Nutrition.* Dec 2022;152(12):2877−88.

[18] Wu G. Dietary protein intake and human health. *Food Funct.* 2016 Mar;7(3):1251−65. doi: 10.1039/c5fo01530h.

[19] Weiler M, Hertzler S. et al. Is it time to reconsider the U.S. recommendations for dietary protein and amino acid intake? *Nutrients.* 2023 Feb 6;15(4):838.

[20] Coelho-Junior H, Marzetti E, et al. Protein intake and frailty: A matter of quantity, quality, and timing. *Nutrients.* 2020;12:2915.

[21] Tomosugi N, Yamamoto S, et al. Effect of collagen tripeptide on atherosclerosis in healthy humans. *J Atheroscler Thromb.* 2017 May 1; 24(5):530−8.

After you eat collagen-rich foods, your body absorbs their specific peptides into your bloodstream. Some of the peptides and amino acids are fuel for the gut lining too. Your body stores a LOT of collagen too. Believe it or not, collagen is about one-third of your body's protein reserves, and it is the most abundant protein type in the body. This means that an immense amount of the protein in your body goes to making collagen.

Collagen has many benefits for digestion. It is nutritious, can reduce inflammation, help heal the gut lining, and may reduce inflammatory bowel disease and IBS; it also helps prevent ulcers and digest foods. Impressively, collagen contains nineteen types of amino acids that are building blocks for the gut lining and for the whole body. These include hydroxyproline, which is found exclusively in collagen. Collagen is also rich in gut-healing amino acids, including glycine, alanine, aspartic acid, glutamic acid, proline, and hydroxyproline.

Did You Know . . . Contrary to Popular Belief, Fat Is a Heart-Protector

For decades, Americans have been told to avoid foods with skin-on and bone-in due to their higher fat content. Yet the collagen in these foods interestingly decreases cholesterol levels, according to some research.[22] It even makes people leaner, which is good for heart health.[23] A recent study even shows

---

[22] Zdzieblik D, Jendricke P, et al. The influence of specific bioactive collagen peptides on body composition and muscle strength in middle-aged, untrained men: A randomized controlled trial. *Int J Environ Res Public Health.* 2021 Apr 30;18(9):4837.

[23] Meroño T, Zamora-Ros R, et al. Animal protein intake is inversely associated with mortality in older adults: The InCHIANTI study. *J Gerontol A Biol Sci Med Sci.* 2022 Sep 1; 77(9):1866–72.

that more animal-based foods protect the heart. [24] [25] [26] While not every research study agrees, we have been led astray from getting gut-healing compounds like collagen. And no, there are no plant-based collagen sources, so if you are vegetarian, you can't get collagen from your diet. This isn't to say that you need to chow down on meat, but the vilification of eating whole animal foods that is popular in the media today is perhaps more harmful than helpful.

About 13 percent of your body's collagen comprises hydroxyproline, found only in collagen-rich foods. This should be enough to consider taking collagen if you don't eat much. Your body makes hydroxyproline more efficiently if you also have a good amount of vitamin C in your diet.

A compound called chondroitin sulfate found in collagen helps prevent leaky gut and prevents unhealthy bacteria from entering the bloodstream from the gut lining. Fascinatingly, it also reduces joint pain in osteoarthritis. If that weren't enough, collagen also is rich in glutamic acid, which helps make glutamine. Glutamine is an amino acid that functions as an antioxidant in the body and helps seal the gut lining. The glutamic acid from collagen has gut-healing properties. It acts as the most essential fuel source for intestinal cells.

As glutamic acid can form glutamate in the gut, it is also a signaling compound that helps coordinate the gut's muscle movements. Glutamine from collagen has many gut health benefits. It reduces intestinal permeability and strengthens the gut lining because it is rich in the amino acid glycine. Glycine increases the production of proteins in the gut called tight junction proteins. So when it comes to leaky gut, collagen is an obvious choice to help heal. This compound also helps improve sleep quality, which is good for the

[24] Bertrand J, Ghouzali I, et al. Glutamine restores tight junction protein claudin-1 expression in colonic mucosa of patients with diarrhea-predominant irritable bowel syndrome. *JPEN J Parenter Enteral Nutr.* 2016 Nov;40(8):1170–6.

[25] Tomé D. The roles of dietary glutamate in the intestine. *Ann Nutr Metab.* 2018;73 Suppl 5:15–20.

[26] Zhou Q, Verne M, et al. Randomised placebo-controlled trial of dietary glutamine supplements for postinfectious irritable bowel syndrome. *Gut.* 2019 Jun;68(6):996–1002.

gut and overall health. Additionally, some research shows that glutamine may reduce small intestinal bacterial overgrowth and reduce IBS. [27] [28]

Did You Know . . . Collagen Is a Natural Anti-Inflammatory

An impressive fact that most people don't know about collagen is that it has natural anti-inflammatory properties. In fact, glycine from collagen helps reduce inflammation which is helpful for the gut and the whole body. This means that collagen may help various health conditions, such as gut issues and joint health. For example, collagen levels are low in people with inflammatory bowel diseases (IBD) such as Crohn's disease and ulcerative colitis.

Bovine collagen contains two gut-healing compounds: hyaluronic acid, which comprises n-acetylglucosamine, and glucuronic acid. The amino acid glycine from collagen helps the body make bile in the liver. Bile is necessary for digestive function because it allows you to absorb fat and vitamins. Glycine from collagen may also protect the liver and help reduce the risk of heart disease.

You know now that collagen helps heal the gut lining. By doing so, collagen helps to increase immune tolerance. By providing healthy protein and gut-healing amino acids, collagen provides building blocks for the immune system as well. It also helps make up the innate immune system by supporting the gut-associated lymphoid tissue.

[27] McBurney M, Yu E, et al. Suboptimal serum α-tocopherol concentrations observed among younger adults and those depending exclusively upon food sources, NHANES 2003-20061-3. *PLoS One.* 2015 Aug 19;10(8):e0135510.

[28] Traber. M. Vitamin E inadequacy in humans: Causes and consequences. *Adv Nutr.* 2014 Sep;5(5):503–14.

Preventing Disease with Vitamin E

At least 90 percent of us don't eat enough vitamin E, even at the paltry **RDI** levels of 20 mg daily.[29] [30] This data comes from the vast numbers of people in the United States, so it is likely an accurate representation of a global problem.

Did You Know . . . Vitamin E Deficiency Is Related to Other Health Issues

A recent study published in the *American Journal of Clinical Nutrition* showed that as many as one in three adults with diabetes or metabolic syndrome have vitamin E deficiency. And 33 percent of obese and overweight adults have an undiagnosed vitamin E deficiency.[31] [32] This puts them at risk for other diseases, including gut malaise. Overweight people likely need more vitamin E due to having more fat tissue, which is easily oxidized or damaged. Vitamin E helps reduce this damage, but the requirements for vitamin E increase the heavier you are.

Diseases that increase the risk of vitamin E deficiency include digestive disorders, cystic fibrosis, cirrhosis, gallbladder disease or removal, obesity, and metabolic syndrome. Drugs that rob the body of vitamin E include cholesterol medicines, laxatives, and antibiotics. In other words, if you suffer from a chronic health condition or take some types of common medications, your odds of vitamin E deficiency are high.

---

[29] Traber M, Mah, E, et al. Metabolic syndrome increases dietary α-tocopherol requirements as assessed using urinary and plasma vitamin E catabolites: A double-blind, crossover clinical trial. *Am J Clin Nutr.* 2017;105(3):571–9.

[30] Borel P, Desmarchelier C. Genetic variations associated with vitamin A status and vitamin A bioavailability. *Nutrients.* 2017 Mar 8;9(3):246.

[31] Ferraro P, Taylor E, , et al. Vitamin B6 intake and the risk of incident kidney stones. *Urolithiasis.* 2018 Jun;46(3):265–70

[32] Durrani D, Idrees R, et al. Vitamin B6: A new approach to lowering anxiety, and depression? *Ann Med Surg (Lond).* 2022 Sep 15;82:104663.

Vitamin E likely helps protect the intestinal wall from damage, so it is vital for gut health. Low levels of vitamin E also likely cause changes in the health of gut bacteria. Luckily, most high-quality multivitamin and minerals supplements contain at least the daily **RDI** of vitamin E.

Activated Vitamin A Is Key

More than ever, we are low in vitamin A and don't know it. The media, even postgraduate nutrition programs, have convinced us that eating carrots and orange vegetables and fruits supplies an abundant amount of vitamin A. For many people, this is misguided because carrots contain beta-carotene, not vitamin A. While some beta carotene can be converted to vitamin A, this is highly dictated by your genes. Over 40 percent of the population are very inefficient at making a carrot into vitamin A,[33] in other words, due to their genetic predisposition. I'm pretty sure most of us haven't studied our genetic profiles in detail. I have and know that my body can't take a carrot and make it into gold, so to speak.

Additionally, the push toward plant-based diets has led us further away from getting active vitamin A. While there is nothing wrong with eating carrots because they are healthy, for some people, this message is disastrous. This is because vitamin A is paramount to a healthy immune response in the gut, partly due to helping maintain a healthy microbiome. Activated vitamin A also helps protect tissues in the gut from inflammatory compounds. People with low vitamin A status have a compromised gut lining which can cause unwanted compounds to enter the bloodstream. This causes the whole body to be under threat of toxins and germs.

Additionally, low-fat diets and restricting cholesterol have made us bypass some of the healthiest foods—organ meats, which are by far the richest sources of vitamin A in the food supply.

---

[33] Park S, Kang S, et al. Folate and vitamin B-12 deficiencies additively impair memory function and disturb the gut microbiota in amyloid-β infused rats. *Int J Vitam Nutr Res.* 2022 Jul;92(3–4):169–81.

It would seem like getting enough vitamin A should be an easy fix. Eat some grass-fed beef liver every week, and all will be well. But this is a tricky fix for some people to swallow, so vitamin A supplements can be a helpful add-in.

Advisory: When to Avoid Supplements

Certain people should avoid high doses of vitamin and mineral supplements. People who are pregnant or have cancer have special nutrient requirements and should avoid taking high doses of certain nutrients. While some of these conditions may benefit from higher amounts of certain nutrients than the **RDI** provides, such as vitamin D3, you should always check with your healthcare provider before adding supplements above the **RDI** for pregnancy or cancer.

B-Vitamins for Gut Maintenance and Why We Are Low

It happens. You may eat a typical American or a fad diet, as people do. Whether it is too much sugar or processed foods, or an overly restrictive diet, there is one thing you should know: these foods and patterns cause your body to burn through your B-vitamin supply. And your gut and the whole body suffers as a result.

Each B vitamin has a slightly different role in the body, but they all are involved in energy transformation. This energy is required for cells to function correctly, including the cells of your gut lining. For example, vitamin B1, thiamine, is necessary for the early steps of turning carbohydrates into energy in the body. Refined carbohydrates in the diet often lack vitamin B1, putting you into a vitamin B1 deficit. These nutrients aren't recycled in the body; you need a constant supply.

So as you slowly become robbed of thiamine by sugar or processed foods, your gut suffers. This is because a lack of thiamine causes your immune system to struggle and thereby reduces your gut-associated immune function. Like thiamine, vitamins B6, B2, B3, and other B vitamins are negatively affected by the typical foods on grocery store shelves today. If that weren't enough, processed foods cause a disruption of the healthy bacteria in the gut. These bacteria not only keep your immune system healthy, but they also can produce some B vitamins like B2 (riboflavin).

Did You Know . . . Processing Robs Grains of Vitamin B

A disease called pellagra first appeared in the late 1700s in Spain and Italy. This was soon after the introduction of corn into their diets. Unless corn is processed with lime to liberate its nutrients, it can cause this condition. Corn became a big part of their diet in these regions and resulted in widespread pellagra. Then again, in the 1900s, pellagra was an epidemic in the United States. The widespread deficiency was related to the processing of grain, which robs it of niacin. Symptoms include abdominal pain, appetite loss, diarrhea, inflamed gut lining, and confusion. Eventually, people die of this condition. While some processed foods add in niacin to a degree, this is an example of how processed foods are very unhealthy and make your gut unhealthy.

B vitamin deficiency is much more common than once thought as well. Diets, alcohol, commonly used medications, and stress can rob you of these critical gut-healing nutrients.

Low levels of vitamin B6 are related to the severity of IBS, and its deficiency is caused by the same pitfalls as other nutrients. Fascinatingly, vitamin B6 reduces inflammation, protects brain health, may help with depression, may even lower cancer risk, and reduce kidney stones when you choose the correct form.[34] We will get into that more in Chapter 6.

Niacin, also known as vitamin B3, helps to reduce premature aging and has anti-aging functions throughout the body. In the gut, it plays these critical roles as well as this regenerative nutrient helps protect the gut lining from

---

[34] Watcharanon W, Kaewrudee S, et al. Effects of sunlight exposure and vitamin D supplementation on vitamin D levels in postmenopausal women in rural Thailand: A randomized controlled trial. *Complement Ther Med.* 2018 Oct;40:243−7.

damaging toxins.

Did You Know . . . Crohn's Disease Can Lead to Niacin Deficiency

An example of a disease state today that leads to niacin deficiency is Crohn's disease. Other conditions that may reduce the body's ability to generate energy from niacin include immunosuppressants, Sinemet, and long-term kidney dialysis. If you have a niacin deficiency, it is almost always worsened by shortages of other vitamins and minerals. And you should know that multiple B-vitamin deficiencies almost always occur together.

A lack of folate, also known as vitamin B9, causes damage to your DNA and can also damage the intestinal lining. This makes absorbing other nutrients difficult and results in inflammation. Research also shows that lacking folate changes the microbiome for the worst.[35] Lacking fresh greens, whole eggs, and organ meats in the diet is a common culprit of folate deficiency.

While these are just some examples of how a lack of various B vitamins negatively affects the gut, you should know that there are many more. This is why most of us benefit from natural B vitamins, and we will delve deeper into this topic in Chapter 6.

The Essential Role of Vitamin C

Vitamin C is an essential nutrient that surprisingly can be missing for many. And the amount of vitamin C established by the RDA has little to do with the amount that will keep your gut healthy. It was established to prevent scurvy, not optimize health.

One primary reason that vitamin C status can be disrupted is if you have low stomach acid levels. Stomach acid medications like **proton pump inhibitors**

---

[35] Moretti H, Colucci V, et al, Vitamin D_3 repletion versus placebo as adjunctive treatment of heart failure patient quality of life and hormonal indices: A randomized, double-blind, placebo-controlled trial. *BMC Cardiovasc Disord.* 2017 Oct 30;17(1):274.

or PPIS (i.e., omeprazole) prevent vitamin C from being absorbed. Being deficient in vitamin C can contribute to inflammation in the gut, which then disrupts the health of the gut lining.

Various health issues can affect your vitamin C status, including body weight, pregnancy and lactation, genetic variants, smoking, and disease states, including severe infections and various non-communicable diseases such as cardiovascular disease and cancer. If you are exposed to secondhand smoke, you are much more likely to have vitamin C deficiency, for example. And if you have a high BMI, you may also have a deficiency in vitamin C.

In other words, vitamin C deficiency is relatively common, contrary to old ways of thinking. Vitamin C helps the body make collagen (see above), reduces inflammation, and has more gut health benefits by being a natural antihistamine when you have higher amounts of it.

Compelling Evidence for the Role of Vitamin D

One nutrient that has compelling influences on the whole body, including your gut, is vitamin D—both a nutrient and hormone. It is essential for the normal functioning of every cell in your body and brain.

Known as the sunshine vitamin, D3 comes mainly from the sun's midday rays or ultraviolet B. Most people don't get enough vitamin D from the sun due to seasonal changes, sun-blocking practices, or living in colder climates.

Vitamin D is also found in small amounts in foods like wild salmon, other oily fish, liver, grass-fed meats, and mushrooms. Food manufacturers also sprinkle a bit into foods like milk and cereals. But, it is next to impossible to get enough vitamin D from food sources alone.

As a potent immune regulator, vitamin D helps your body's natural immune defenses by making antimicrobial compounds. Your gut is home to most of your immune system, so vitamin D has countless roles in protecting it and your gut. Impressively, vitamin D even helps regulate genes.

Vitamin D deficiency is even related to cancer risk, heart disease risk, diabetes risk, spinal stenosis, headaches, and low back pain, to name a few conditions. But, there are common roadblocks and misconceptions about getting vitamin D in the diet and supplements. Milk drinkers think they are fine when their milk only contains a drop-in-the-bucket amount of how much vitamin D they need. Some people also feel like they get sun exposure, so their vitamin D levels should be acceptable. Yet, a study of sun exposure over twelve weeks wasn't enough to restore blood levels of vitamin D for women living in Thailand.[36] However, sun AND supplements increased blood levels to a normal range.

Other people feel they take a daily multivitamin, so they should be covered. But most supplements contain only 400 IU, insufficient to budge your vitamin D levels unless you are a small child. And desk-job workers are notoriously low in vitamin D. This is because the sun angles at 5 or 6 p.m. in the northern hemisphere are too oblique to give you enough vitamin D when you get off of work.

Did You Know . . .Vitamin D Is Vital for Heart Health

I helped facilitate a research project using vitamin D treatment in heart failure patients. We found that vitamin D supplementation at 10,000 IU per day for six months improved the quality of life and function of people with heart failure. These patients also had improved lab values that are surrogate markers of outcomes, such as C-reactive protein.[37] While research is still considered early in this area, the results from a compilation of 465 patients showed improved heart failure outcomes with doses greater than 4000 IU of vitamin D per day.

Vitamin D substantially decreases some of the most significant inflammatory components in the gut, including NF-kB. Multiple research studies show that vitamin D can change the ratio of T cells, improving T- regulatory

36 Mocanu V, Oboroceanu T, et al. Current status in vitamin D and regulatory T cells—immunological implications. *Rev Med Chir Soc Med Nat Iasi.* 2013 Oct–Dec; 117(4):965–73.

37 Montgomery D, Biklé A, et al. Soil health and nutrient density: Preliminary comparison of regenerative and conventional farming. *PeerJ.* 2022;10:e12848.

cells and preventing the body from attacking itself. [38] This is why vitamin D likely help prevent or help treat gut conditions related to immune issues like Crohn's disease, ulcerative colitis, and more. Moreover, because vitamin D acts as a hormone, it influences thousands of bodily functions. It has even been shown in some case reports of children with enlarged hearts to help normalize heart function.

Did You Know . . . It's Easy to Test Your Vitamin D Levels

Vitamin D can easily be checked at home using a variety of at-home test kits. Their accuracy is often as good or better than most labs in medical facilities and can save you money compared to hospital-based labs. The quality criteria for these tests are easy to spot on the label. Examples of reputable companies offering at-home vitamin D test kits are Grassroots Health, Imaware, and Everlywell. Aim for a vitamin D level of around 40–60 ng/ml as this is ideal, but some people optimize their health at higher levels of vitamin D than this.

When buying vitamin D test kits online, look for the following criteria:

- Liquid chromatography/mass spectrometry testing
- Clinical Laboratory Improvement Amendments (CLIA) Approved
- Total 25-hydroxyvitamin D levels

The Multiple Roles of Vitamin K

Once thought to be the clotting vitamin, vitamin K also plays complex, essential roles in the health of your brain, gut, bones, and heart. In fact, certain kinds of vitamin K—called menaquinones or vitamin K2—may even help prevent and reverse aspects of heart disease and other health problems.

Not surprisingly, vitamin K helps support a healthy and robust microbiome too. It likely helps dampen gut inflammation, increase beneficial bacteria,

---

[38] Mocanu V, Oboroceanu T, et al. Current status in vitamin D and regulatory T cells— immunological implications. *Rev Med Chir Soc Med Nat Iasi.* 2013 Oct–Dec; 117(4):965–73.

reduce toxins like lipopolysaccharides, and even prevent excess clotting. Vitamin K also is critical for helping to maintain adequate vitamin D (see above) levels in the body by increasing vitamin D receptors.

However, not all vitamin K is the same. Vitamin K1 from leafy greens is a weaker form than K2 in natto, a fermented soybean paste, grass-finished meats, and butter. Still, eating both kinds is essential: vitamin K1 from leafy greens and vitamin K2 from natto and grass-finished meats. However, most people don't eat natto, much less know what it is. Some estimates show that between 50–97 percent of the population is low in vitamin K2, including children. And it's difficult and expensive to get grass-finished meats for many people. So, supplemental vitamin K2 can be a helpful addition to most people's diets.

Gut Disruptors—Antinutrients

If you think plants want to be eaten, you are wrong. Plants have built-in protective compounds that upset the gut, so you avoid eating them again. Some of these compounds are called **antinutrients**. These compounds cause irritation in the gut lining and poor nutrient absorption. Antinutrients in foods include tannins, phytic acid, lectins, saponins, trypsin inhibitors, oxalates, and even healthy antioxidant compounds called polyphenols that act to reduce nutrient absorption. While some of these compounds can have some of their own health benefits, the amounts of them and the health of your gut dictate whether or not they will go over well when you eat them.

Over time we have become quite adept at working around these antinutrients by learning to cook and prepare them properly, such as fermenting and soaking them. Some foods like corn require an extensive process called nixtamalization or processing with an alkali solution and carefully grinding to remove the hull.

Sadly, our fast-paced world doesn't usually stop us from preparing foods like our ancestors did to reduce these antinutrients. You may have experienced this if you have ordered a burrito at a restaurant. I can guarantee that the beans were not appropriately prepared to remove the antinutrients in the beans or corn. So you are left with a hot mess in your gut, so to speak. If there is one food that consistently causes upset bellies, it is beans in fast-paced restaurants.

The other culprit is gluten grains, which contain a host of antinutrients and gut-disrupting aspects. Gluten sensitivity and intolerance are increasing issues for many of us. The cause of high rates of gluten intolerance is unknown but is likely due to many factors. For example, there is more gluten in each grain of wheat today due to hybridization and could also be related to the high amounts of glyphosate used. It is likely also partially related to the fact that wheat is no longer fermented as it was in times gone by, such as in sourdough bread and fermented grains. Last but not least, the human gut is exposed to many antibiotics, which sets us up to have more food allergies and sensitivities, including gluten.

Even quinoa is rife with antinutrients too called saponins. Most people don't prepare quinoa well, so it can also be a gut-disruptive food at times. While eating certain plants can and should be a part of a healthy diet, it should be done with the care and respect it deserves. After all, they don't want to be eaten and will do everything to keep you from being consumed in the future for their own survival.

Fiber in Gut Health

Talking about antinutrients leads us to the so-called mainstay of gut health—fiber. The problem is there are so many kinds that it isn't fair to put them all in the same category. Each plant's skeletal system is made of unique fibers, and if you haven't noticed, plants are very complex and different. For example, I would never think of the pectin fiber from an apple as the fiber from wheat bran. Each fiber-rich food needs to be looked at from its own holistic perspective.

An excellent example of this is flax seeds. Each blossom of a flax flower produces four to ten seeds. Gathering flax seeds in a traditional diet would have produced a relatively small amount of these seeds. In other words, I don't believe that the human body was meant to eat many of these at one time.

My experience with flax fiber is that it can be one of the most gut-painful foods, especially if it isn't fermented. So yes, while rich in fiber, it, like other fibrous foods, needs careful consideration.

You can suffer from a low-fiber diet because of the modern pitfalls discussed earlier in the chapter. And fiber would seem like a straightforward win for gut health. It can help, but the problem is fiber can be one of the most daunting ingredients in the diet because it hitchhikes with the antinutrients such as phytic acid. As you may recall, these antinutrients bind nutrients, making them unavailable to the body. In other words, if it isn't fermented, it can upset your gut. I would never recommend getting fiber from wheat bran or granola, or quick-processed beans, in other words.

Still, certain types of fibers are gentler on the body and can help certain gut conditions, especially IBS, diarrhea, and constipation, when chosen wisely and introduced slowly. Generally, acacia fiber, psyllium, guar gum, and pectin fibers are the best to add as supplements.

The Role of Minerals

You probably know that conventional foods have more chemical residues than organically or regeneratively grown foods. But, what you may not know is that standard farming practices have continually drained the soil of its ability to transfer nutrients like minerals to the food it grows in. As I shared with you earlier in this chapter (see page 14), the soil's microbiome suffers from conventional farming and ranching, which makes the planet and you suffer if it isn't grown in a way that nature intends it to.

For example, regeneratively farmed cabbage has 50 percent more zinc and magnesium than the amounts listed in the USDA Nutrient Database.[39] Not to mention 70 percent more **antioxidant**-rich compounds called phenolics than vegetables found in typical New York supermarkets. And wheat grown in no-till ways had about a third to a half more minerals like zinc and magnesium.

---

[39] Montgomery D, Biklé A, et al. Soil health and nutrient density: Preliminary comparison of regenerative and conventional farming. *PeerJ.* 2022;10:e12848.

Strikingly, conventionally grown foods had substantially more unwanted heavy metals such as cadmium and nickel than regeneratively grown foods in these studies.[40]

You should know that it is challenging to find regeneratively grown foods most of the time, but your odds are better if you shop for produce and meats at local farmer's markets. The extra time and effort are worth it for your health. Processed foods and prescriptions can also deplete your mineral stores or make it harder to absorb them from your diet, so supplemental minerals make a lot of sense.

So, having looked at all the nutrition we need for glorious gut health, the question is, how do we make up for the years of nutrient depletion? You will learn more about this in Chapter 6; for now, let's move on to the world of supplements.

---

[40] Mayo Clinic. Are organic foods worth the price? *Mayo Clinic, Mayo Foundation for Medical Education and Research.* 2022 Apr 22. https://www.mayoclinic.org/healthy-lifestyle/nutritio n-and-healthy-eating/in-depth/organic-food/art-20043880.

4

Chapter 4

What's in the Bottle: Choosing Supplements

Most supplements have a reasonably long track record of safety, but there are some individual concerns you should consider for your unique needs. In this chapter, you will learn why natural medicines disappeared from conventional medical practice, issues with supplement regulations, which supplements to avoid, precautions for taking certain supplements, and how to find the best supplements.

Why Natural Medicine Disappeared

Many people don't realize that herbal and natural medicines were primarily banned from being taught in medical schools due to the single-handed ambitions of Abraham Flexner, the author of the 1910 Flexner Report.[41]

---

[41] Stahnisch F, Verhoef M. The Flexner report of 1910 and its impact on complementary and alternative medicine and psychiatry in North America in the 20th century. *Evid Based Complement Alternat Med.* 2012;2012:647896.

Flexner was a teacher, not a doctor, and was hired by the Carnegie Foundation, which had much to gain by helping spearhead Big Pharma.[42] Due to Flexner's persuasive report, plant medicine vanished from medical schools, and those teaching herbal medicine were shut down by 1930 on the strength of Flexner's recommendation.

For this reason, herbs and natural remedies as medicine are a lost art for most healthcare practitioners now. The science of natural medicine remains largely neglected even when there have been good research studies evaluating them in recent years. [43] This is also very strange because many cancer drugs are derived from plants! Natural medicine research goes undiscovered due to several reasons. One big factor is that there is a lack of dissemination of information on herbs because medical journals today are heavily funded by Big Pharma. The most commonly read medical journals by physicians are also implicated in passing over natural medicine research in favor of publishing papers about drugs that further their Big Pharma agenda.

But a good example of the vast extent of research on natural medicine is to look at the National Library of Medicine. For turmeric alone, over 7,000 publications about the research-backed benefits of its various uses have been published and are available on this research database. But, established dogma and funneling of resources in medicine today are almost exclusively dedicated to pharmaceuticals. So unless you are a sleuth for finding information about health topics, research on herbs and natural medicine is rarely found, let alone disseminated to doctors.

My mission is to help you find natural medicines to support your gut health despite all the obstacles.

---

[42] The Influence of The Carnegie Foundation on Medical Education. *JAMA.* 1909;LIII(7):559–60.

[43] Turmeric - Search Results - Pubmed. National Center for Biotechnology Information, U.S. National Library of Medicine. https://pubmed.ncbi.nlm.nih.gov/?term=turmeric.

What About Supplement Regulation?

A concern often raised in the media regards the regulation of natural supplements and natural medicines. But let's explore if regulation helps at all in other situations. Let's look at the regulation of food labeling, for example. The American Heart Association (AHA) has created a heart symbol for packaged food labels complying with their specific regulations. If a food is low in saturated fat, low in sodium, and has modest amounts of a nutrient, i.e., fiber, it can have the AHA heart symbol on it, which signals to the public that this food is indeed healthy. But sweetened soy milk loaded with added refined sugar gets the heart symbol, while a wholesome egg doesn't make the cut.[44] These regulations and guidelines can mislead us into eating more packaged and processed foods because they are approved as "heart healthy." But the rise in obesity and chronic disease is related to some processed foods, including ultra-processed foods like sweetened soy milk, according to the *British Journal of Nutrition*.[45]

Another example of failed regulations is the so-called safe over-the-counter medications. Digestive medications like PPIs (proton pump inhibitors) are available to anyone. They are often taken copiously with little regard for their potential to damage health, including an increased risk of heart disease, bone loss, dementia, and more.[46] Regulated medications like these, along with many others, cause infinitely more harm than most supplements.

---

[44] Heart.org. Heart-check food certification program. https://www.heart.org/-/media/Health y-Living-Files/Heart-Check-files/Monthly-Grocery-List-2022/Heart_Check_Certified_ Products_010522.pdf

[45] Pagliai G, Dinu M, et al. Consumption of ultra-processed foods and health status: A systematic review and meta-analysis. *Br J Nutr.* 2021 Feb 14;125(3):308-18. doi: 10.1017/S0007114520002688. Epub 2020 Aug 14. PMID: 32792031; PMCID: PMC7844609.

[46] Yibirin M, De Oliveira D, et al. Adverse effects associated with proton pump inhibitor use. *Cureus.* 2021 Jan 18;13(1):e12759.

Safety Issues

Most supplements are safe, and negative issues are much less risky than many prescription and over-the-counter drugs. For example, research shows that the main reason someone goes to the emergency room (ER) for supplement use is due to a choking incident or swallowing issues in the elderly or overdosing on supplements for weight loss. The total number of ER visits due to supplements annually is around 20,000 incidents in the United States.[47] In contrast, about 20 percent of all ER visits, close to six million annually, are attributable to prescription medication errors and overuse.[48]

The supplements that are usually best avoided are those used to rapidly increase exercise performance and muscle gain. While some of them have been banned in the United States, it is still possible to get them shipped from overseas. Along with weight-loss supplements, these generally hold a higher risk than others. Additionally, **synthetic vitamins that come with longer-term risks** are to be generally avoided.

So let's look at why.

Stimulants

If you want to support your gut health, logically, you should limit stimulants in general (that includes caffeine, alcohol, and other recreational drugs). Stimulants can cause anxiety which is most often felt in the gut. Excess caffeine, use of ephedra, and energy drink powders are some things to avoid.

Ginseng is technically stimulating, as are some medicinal mushrooms. Still, they have their own set of benefits for gut health and may even help reduce anxiety, so this is an exception to the rule.

---

[47] Geller A, Shehab N, et al. Emergency department visits for adverse events related to dietary supplements. *N Engl J Med.* 2015 Oct 15;373(16):1531–40.

[48] Nymoen L, Björk M, et al. Drug-related emergency department visits: prevalence and risk factors. *Intern Emerg Med.* 2022; 17:1453–62.

Natural Steroids

There are supplements on the market today that can naturally help balance hormones, but these should not be taken without monitoring by your healthcare provider. Examples to generally avoid in this category are DHEA and androstenedione.

Synthetic Vitamins

Vitamins in their natural forms usually work better than synthetic vitamins because the body uses them more effectively and retains them better. I will explain how they work better than synthetic vitamins in the next paragraphs. While many vitamins can be made cheaply in a factory, they are often slightly different than their natural counterparts. This difference in chemical composition makes it so the body is often unable to use them effectively. They can even cause damage to your health in some cases.

For example, natural folate is better than folic acid—a synthetic vitamin. Recent research shows that a common **gene variant** called MTHFR makes folic acid supplements problematic for many people because they can block folate receptors in the body, leaving unmetabolized folic acid in the bloodstream.[49]

The long-term health consequences of this are not fully understood, but people with MTHFR gene variants, which is around half of the population, do not get any benefit from taking folic acid. In fact, some studies show that folic acid, in this case, is linked to preterm births, increased cancer risk, nausea, irritability, and more. Better choices of folate for anyone are naturally sourced and are listed on labels as natural folate, L-MTHF (l-methyltetrahydrofolate), folinic acid, levomefolate, calcium folinate, and methylfolate.

Other synthetic vitamins you should generally avoid:

---

[49] Shah M, Murad W, et al. Multiple health benefits of curcumin and its therapeutic potential. *Environ Sci Pollut Res Int.* 2022 Jun;29(29):43732–44.

- dl-alpha-tocopherol (synthetic vitamin E
- pyridoxine (synthetic vitamin B6)
- cyanocobalamin (synthetic vitamin B12)

There are many brands on the market today that you might think are natural but are not, including:

- Flintstones multivitamins
- One-A-Day multivitamins
- Centrum multivitamins
- Nature Made multivitamins
- Store brands like Kirkland/Equate vitamins and Mega Food multivitamins (there may still be some quality products within these brands, but their multivitamins contain many undesirable ingredients)

Advisory: Medication Interactions

If your prescribed medication interacts negatively with a particular supplement, you should avoid it. An excellent example of this is that vitamin K interacts with warfarin. There are ways to take it, but you must be monitored and disclose that you are taking it to your healthcare provider. Another example is grapefruit extract, which needs to be avoided with many medications. While these are a couple examples of significant drug interactions, there are others that you need to closely discuss with your pharmacist and healthcare provider.

That said, there are often positive interactions with supplements and medications. An excellent example of this is when you take statins or cholesterol drugs. Taking vitamin D, vitamin K, coenzyme Q10, and other supplements can be really helpful in reducing some of the side effects of the medications. In other words, you can't assume that there are adverse interactions with your medicines because, more often than not, supplements make up for the nutrients that medications deplete.

Supplement Sensitivities

Food sensitivities are pretty common, which can also be true of supplements. So the cardinal rule here is that if you don't feel good when you take something, even if generally considered healthy, avoid it.

An excellent example is turmeric. For most people, supplementing turmeric is beneficial because it dampens inflammation, reduces cancer risk, helps improve gut health, and more.[50] However, some people feel worse when they take it.

Some supplements contain common allergens, too, like soy, corn, wheat, and dairy. If you know you are allergic or sensitive to these foods, read the labels of any supplements to make sure they are free of foods that cause you to feel bad.

That said, most supplements can make you feel off if you don't take them with food, so that can be an easy fix. Common sense should tell you to avoid any risk of choking, always take supplements with water, and don't swallow handfuls at a time.

Choosing Supplements

Choosing the best forms of supplements can help you get more out of the supplements you buy and helps your body absorb these supplements more efficiently too. There are a vast array of supplements on the market, and the following guidelines can help you choose the best ones.

Avoid Tablets

Regarding supplements, there are so many forms on the market today. Generally speaking, gel caps, powders, and capsules are well-absorbed by the body and are often free of fillers and additives. In contrast, tablet

[50] Pfeiffer C, Sternberg M, et al. Unmetabolized folic acid is detected in nearly all serum samples from US children, adolescents, and adults. *J Nutr.* 2015 Mar;145(3):520–31.

supplements always have unwanted **fillers** and are often much more poorly absorbed. Tablet forms are not the same quality, and low-quality vitamins are almost always in tablet form.

Look for Third-Party Certification

The best supplements can be hard to distinguish from low-quality brands because all vitamin companies want to sell their product to you. No wonder the supplement aisles and online stores are confusing; there are just so many options.

For the best vitamin and supplement brands, certification of quality, potency, and purity is essential. You can look for GMP (Good Manufacturing Practices) on your label to know if your supplement has what it says it has. GMP-certified vitamin supplements are consistently high in quality, and help guarantee pure products because they are checked for quality by independent third-party companies.

NSF International is a company that often conducts third-party testing to ensure that vitamin and supplement products meet safety and health standards. You will often see the NSF certification on high-quality supplement labels as well.

A supplement dispensary that you can use that contains all GMP-certified products, and all products are also considered pharmaceutical grade is Fullscript. You can find a natural healthcare practitioner with one of these accounts or use mine: https://us.fullscript.com/welcome/hmoretti/. Disclosure: I make a small affiliate income if you use this link.

Choose Activated Vitamin Forms

Activated vitamins are usually the best option for health because they don't rely on the body's enzymes to efficiently convert into ideal forms of vitamins. An excellent example of this is activated folate or activated B6 as pyridoxal-5-phosphate. Other examples of activated vitamins are vitamin D3, a better form of vitamin D than vitamin D2. Ironically, prescription vitamin D2 contains the less-desirable form called vitamin D2. Another example of an activated vitamin is retinol palmitate, which is preferable over beta-carotene because around 40 percent of us don't efficiently make active vitamin A from plant sources.[51]

Select Capsules, Gelcaps, Chewables, and Powders

Simply put, capsules, chewable and liquid vitamins are easier for the body to break down than tablets. They are also much easier to swallow. With tablet vitamin forms, much of it may go directly into the toilet, unfortunately.

Capsules are also less likely to be full of filler ingredients, and chewable vitamins are great for children because they are easier to swallow.

Avoid gummy vitamins for adults and children because while they may taste good, they are generally very lacking! The exception for gummies is when you want to take extra vitamin C or extra vitamin D. In this case, taking a gummy vitamin is fine.

Find Absorbable Minerals

Some forms of minerals in supplements pass through the body without absorbing well, if at all. A supplement brand is only as good as its absorption ability, so it helps to have them in **chelated** forms. I'll explain more.

Minerals like magnesium, zinc, or potassium are attached to **amino acids** or **organic compounds**, which is chelation. Examples of chelated minerals are bound to an amino acid—e.g., magnesium malate, magnesium glycinate, magnesium citrate, iron bisglycinate, and zinc carnosine.

Less absorbable minerals have their place, as is in the case of magnesium oxide if used to help increase the frequency of bowel movements. But, they are less readily absorbed as nutritional magnesium.

---

[51] Suzuki M, Tomita, M. Genetic variations of vitamin A-absorption and storage-related genes, and their potential contribution to vitamin A deficiency risks among different ethnic groups. *Front Nutr.* 2022 Apr 28;9:861619.

The Golden Rules of Supplements

Dietary supplements get a bad name because they can make people feel bad-but they shouldn't if they are of good quality. To summarize, choose supplements that:

- Purchase supplements legally on sale in your country from trustworthy suppliers with good consumer reviews.
- Avoid stimulants, weight-loss, and exercise performance supplements, mainly if they contain stimulants. If you decide to take these supplements, stick to the advised dosage or the lowest possible dose and stop taking them if you notice any adverse reactions.
- Choose supplements that come as capsules, gels, and powders. Avoid tablets and gummy-style supplements.

Many people stop taking supplements because they feel worse when they take them and get stomach pains and discomfort. Synthetic vitamins are usually harsher on the body than natural ones. Low-quality minerals don't absorb well either, leaving your belly with unease. Factory-made vitamins may create intestinal imbalances from additives and chemicals, and the following tips should help you avoid any intestinal side effects:

- Take your supplements with food for better absorption and to help ease your stomach.
- Take your supplements in smaller, more frequent doses, at least twice daily.
- Use the sight-smell test. A herb or vitamin should look and smell like what it is made from.
- Product reviews are essential. The more positive reviews a product has, the better it likely is.
- Whole food compounds hold little or no risk because you would eat them anyway.

5

Chapter 5

Gut Healing Whole Food Supplements

In Chapter 3, you learned all about why your gut might be suffering due to low nutrient intake. In this chapter, you will learn how to be a savvy consumer of whole-food nutritional supplements and extracts to help heal your gut and increase its ability to absorb nutrients more readily.

Unfortunately, the best supplements and nutrition for your body can be expensive and take some planning. It may be the best money you have ever spent because treating the root cause of your gut issues may mean avoiding a prescription drug. But you should always discuss these additions with your healthcare provider, preferably one that has had extensive training in nutrition. I recommend functional medicine doctors, naturopaths, or functional nutritionists.

What Does Your Body Need

For most people, a broad-spectrum multivitamin with minerals, an omega 3 supplement, extra vitamin D3, vitamin K2, and probiotics is a good start, as we will explore in more depth in Chapter 6. For now, let's review whole-food supplements that are helpful for many gut conditions. Don't worry. You will have all of Chapter 7 to learn about herbal supplements for gut healing too.

Read through all of the following supplements to see if any resonate with what your body needs. It is challenging to find reliable brands of whole food products at times, so where there are currently challenges, you'll find some recommendations on page 304. In the following chapters, you will find more specific guidance on when and how to use these supplements for specific gut conditions.

Organ Meats (Including Intestine)

Before you get grossed out by this one, consider where we came from. Humans, before the last century or so ago, never wasted any food, especially not organ meats. This is because our ancestors knew they provided the body with the most nutrient-rich source of foods we could get.

The approach of like-treats-like also comes into play. When we suffer from health problems, our organs often fail. While there are no clinical trials that really prove this, countless practitioners over time, including myself, find that adding organ meats into the diet is a life-changer if done consistently and thoughtfully.

If you add or already eat organ meats, you can probably forgo a lot of other vitamin supplements too. For example, 4 oz of liver meets your needs for vitamin B12, vitamin A, folate, and choline needs for the day. This also provides over half your daily needs for iron, selenium, chromium, and copper. Organ tissues like the heart, liver, and spleen are rich in vitamins, minerals, antioxidants, and healing compounds. For example, the only natural source of an antioxidant called coenzyme Q10 is organ meats, especially the heart. Liver is rich in hyaluronic acid and collagen, too, both building blocks for gut cells.

Like many people, you likely weren't raised to eat organ meats. If you simply can't face eating them regularly, you can find many supplemental forms. Supplementing liver is a good place to start. The only caution is if you have iron overload or Wilson's disease; in these cases, you should avoid taking extra liver, heart, or spleen. Just make sure to choose 100 percent grass-finished organ meats from beef because they are more nutritious and do not contain any harmful inflammatory compounds.

Still skeptical? I encourage you to look at reviews of organ meat supplements and read the comments. They are almost always life-changing for the better for people. For example, on Amazon, there are over 1200 ratings for Ancestral Supplements Intestines supplements (see also page 304). Like-treating-like, people are amazed by it; some say it's the only thing that has EVER helped their digestive issues, while others say it helps bowel movements, mood, focus, reduces inflammation, improves sleep, and more.

You can wait thirty years and hope someone does a clinical trial of organ meats for gut health. Or, because they are super nutritious with minimal to no side effects, you can try them. Personally, I won't ever be without organ meats again because they improved my hormonal and gut health tremendously. But, again, like-treats-like may mean you want to take gallbladder, liver, and intestines. Or you may want to take heart and spleen because of the natural iron source and antioxidants they provide.

Omega-3 Fats

There is no question that most people's diets are too low in healthy omega-3 fats. Remember, this nutrient is vital in promoting a healthy microbiome, dampens inflammation, enhances the endocannabinoid system, and is critical for proper gut-cell functioning.

Sure, you could eat more oily fish to get more omega-3 but do you? The average American doesn't eat enough fish, and I admit I don't either, not by choice but because of cost and picky family members. From healthcare savings, omega-3 supplements pay for themselves many times over for the endless preventive benefits they have on the whole body. But quality and form are essential when choosing your supplement. I recommend cod liver oil and krill oil for almost everyone, and I will explain why next.

Traditionally, people take cod liver oil supplements because it is much richer in vitamin A, antioxidants, and **phospholipids** and is absorbed better than other fish oils. Krill oil is also a good choice because it contains astaxanthin, antioxidants, and **phospholipids** and absorbs better than most common fish oil supplements.

The active vitamin A from cod liver oil is a potent antioxidant. In its active form called retinol, vitamin A is critical for a healthy gut, immune system, healing skin tissue, eye health, memory, regulating genes, and heart health. A good cod liver oil contains 1000–5000 IU of vitamin A per teaspoon or around 20–100 percent of the **RDI**. This is important because vitamin A levels are low for more people than most people realize due to a variety of genes that control beta-carotene absorption. So, many people need active vitamin A from animal sources and don't know it.

Additionally, vitamin A from cod liver oil is absorbed well: around 70–90 percent of vitamin A from cod liver oil is absorbed into your bloodstream. In contrast, only 3 percent of plant forms, such as beta-carotene, are absorbed, on average. When you also consider that most people avoid eating vitamin A-rich foods like beef liver, the case for taking cod liver oil becomes even stronger. In a nutshell, I recommend taking cod liver oil and perhaps alternating it with krill oil to optimize your omega-3 intake and nutrient intake.

Collagen

As you may recall from Chapter 3, collagen helps prevent a leaky gut, dampens inflammation, and overall is healing for the gut. Low collagen levels can appear in many ways: low blood pressure, wrinkles and dry skin, joint pain, gut issues, arthritis symptoms, and bone loss. As we grow older, we all lose collagen too. In fact, some tissues in the body typically have three times more collagen when people are in their twenties than when they are eight years old.

Collagen contains healing amino acids for the stomach lining. Some research even suggests that collagen for acid reflux is helpful. [52] It is unknown whether or not collagen affects stomach acid production, but it likely has an overall protective effect on the stomach. For example, supplemental collagen is rich in amino acids like glycine that help to protect the stomach cells against gastric ulcers. This means that collagen may be helpful for gastritis and GERD. Collagen may even reduce the damaging effects of alcohol on the stomach.

If you don't see yourself eating collagen-rich foods daily, like slow-cooked bone-in meats, chicken skin, bone broth, sardines with the skin, or organ meats, you should consider taking collagen supplements. For gut health, it is ideal to choose a collagen protein supplement that contains Type I, Type II, and Type III collagen peptides.

Colostrum

Colostrum is a compound found in the first milking and is extracted from cow's milk. Cow's milk is exceptionally high in colostrum levels right after a mother gives birth to boost the baby's immunity, and cows make an abundant supply of it. Immune problems are rooted in the gut, and many people who struggle with gut issues lack healing compounds like immunoglobulins. Using colostrum makes a lot of sense for helping to heal the gut because it is rich in protective antibodies, nutrients, lactoferrin, immunoglobulins, growth factors, and other healthy compounds that may help heal a body under stress.

---

[52] Martin K, Emil, S, et al. Dextranomer hyaluronic acid copolymer effects on gastroesophageal junction. J. Pediatr. Gastroenterol. Nutr. 2014;58:593–97.

Did You Know . . . Bovine Colostrum Products Heal Leaky Gut

Several clinical studies demonstrate that bovine colostrum supplements help reduce leaky gut.[53] [54] It also contains supportive digestive enzymes that increase the ability to digest foods. Colostrum even reduces a marker of **leaky gut** called zonulin, which increases the gaps between intestinal cells, resulting in intestinal "leakiness." People taking bovine colostrum experience reduced stool zonulin levels and zonulin blood levels. This is a good thing because it indicates it helps heal the gut.

Amazingly, colostrum is curative for my seasonal and household allergies, which are often rooted in having a leaky gut. My only caution when using colostrum is to avoid it if you have a true milk allergy. It is very low in lactose, so most people can tolerate colostrum just fine.

Glutamine

Immune cells in the gut directly rely on glutamine, an **amino acid**. This is especially true when the body is under stress due to infections, surgery, high-intensity exercise, injuries, and inflammatory conditions in the gut. A high protein diet typically provides up to 3 g of glutamine daily from meats, chicken, bone broth, fish, eggs, nuts, seeds, and legumes. In contrast, the body's pools are about a gram of glutamine per kilogram. So, a person weighing 70 kg would have about 70 g stored in the body. But illnesses and gut issues can quickly put the body in a glutamine deficit.

Glutamine uses are numerous from a functional medicine standpoint because it is a predominant amino acid and has critical roles in the gastrointestinal tract. L-glutamine is the most abundant amino acid in the gut, and a lack of it may cause leaky gut. Intestinal "leakiness" is healed

---

[53] Hałasa M, Maciejewska D, et al. "Oral supplementation with bovine colostrum decreases intestinal permeability and stool concentrations of zonulin in athletes. *Nutrients.* 2017 Apr.

[54] Dziewiecka H, Buttar H, et al. A systematic review of the influence of bovine colostrum supplementation on leaky gut syndrome in athletes: Diagnostic biomarkers and future directions. *Nutrients.* 2022 Jun 17;14(12):2512.

by supplemental glutamine when given to people with intestinal infections. Also, glutamine restores tight junction proteins in the gut, so it makes sense that it may heal leaky gut symptoms. By reducing inflammatory compounds in the gut, glutamine also supports a healthy intestinal lining. It is also the primary energy source for your intestinal cells as well.

Additionally, glutamine may reduce small intestine bacterial overgrowth and reduces harmful bacteria growth in the intestines, according to early research work published in the *World Journal of Gastroenterology*.[55] Irritable bowel symptoms after intestinal infection are alleviated by supplemental glutamine. These symptoms include a reduction in diarrhea and leaky gut. Using it for IBS is safe, and the benefits are self-evident, according to numerous research studies.[56]

The best form of supplemental glutamine is powder, which is easily absorbed and free of unwanted additives. Glutamine with protein powder or protein shakes is not ideal because certain amino acids compete with glutamine for absorption, so I suggest avoiding those. For good gut health, glutamine powders often contain other gut healing compounds, such as zinc, n-acetylglucosamine, slippery elm, or licorice. These are great for a short-term gut healing protocol. In other words, you can usually take glutamine for a short period; most people do not require it for longer than a week.

Take glutamine between meals for the best effectiveness. You can also sip on glutamine before bed. If you take it with meals, the amino acids in your food will compete with the glutamine, making it less effective. If you feel nauseated, try starting it with a small amount of food, such as rice. Try sipping on glutamine powder mixed with a bit of lemon juice. From personal experience, if you consume it throughout the day by taking small sips, it has a better chance of having a continual healing effect on the tight junctions of the intestine.

---

[55] Hałasa M, Maciejewska D, et al. "Oral supplementation with bovine colostrum decreases intestinal permeability and stool concentrations of zonulin in athletes. *Nutrients.* 2017 Apr.

[56] Zhu A. N-Acetylglucosamine for treatment of inflammatory bowel disease–a real-world pragmatic clinical trial. *Natural Medicine Journal.* 2015 April 1.

NAG

One of the most impressive supplements for gut pain is called NAG, short for n-acetylglucosamine. This supplement often remarkably improves IBS and inflammatory bowel conditions. It is the only thing that takes away the pain for some people, in fact.

One of the ways NAG works is by reducing the biofilm on harmful bacteria. Biofilms make bacteria extremely resistant to treatment and make them all the more infectious for bacteria such as E. coli. For this reason, it may be beneficial for conditions like SIBO and other inflammatory bowel conditions.

Did You Know . . . Remarkable Statistics for NAG

In a real-world study, 88 percent of people with inflammatory bowel diseases, such as ulcerative colitis or Crohn's disease, felt relief when taking NAG.[57] [58] This is impressive because drug treatments for these conditions often have some pretty adverse side effects, whereas NAG has no significant side effects.

NAG also has other gut benefits; it reduces stomach bloating and may improve bowel movements to relieve constipation. It may enhance your body's ability to absorb nutrients and increase the protective mucin production in the gut to help reduce inflammation and irritation.

You can get NAG in capsules or powder form, and generally speaking, follow the dosing directions on the package. Because NAG is derived from shellfish, you should avoid NAG if you are allergic to shellfish.

[57] Roxas M. The role of enzyme supplementation in digestive disorders. *Altern Med Rev.* 2008 Dec;13(4):307–14.

[58] Zhu A. N-Acetylglucosamine for treatment of inflammatory bowel disease-a real-world pragmatic clinical trial. *Natural Medicine Journal.* April 1, 2015.

Digestive Enzymes

Digestive enzymes are the compounds that break down food so your body absorbs it. These critical enzymes come from three places: fresh and whole foods, the gut lining, and the pancreas. But let's face it: most of us don't eat enough fresh foods and whole foods, and because of this, we lack the enzymes from foods due to heating and processing. Another reason many people need enzyme supplements is that their guts are inflamed. The lining of the digestive tract makes up a big bulk of enzymes for digestive processes starting in your mouth and ending in your colon. When the gut lining is leaky and not functioning well, you likely aren't making enough digestive enzymes. The pancreas also produces digestive enzymes that provide a significant mealtime bolus of enzymes into your intestines when you eat. But inflammation in the pancreas and bile ducts can reduce your body's ability to get enzymes from here too.

If you have a digestive issue, the odds are that you are also low in enzymes. Lack of enzymes can even show up in other parts of the body due to poor digestion of nutrients. Here are some of the reasons you may be low in digestive enzymes:

- Inflammation of the pancreas due to diabetes
- Processed carbohydrates
- Gallstones
- Gallbladder removal
- Alcohol
- Vitamin or mineral deficiencies
- High-calorie diets
- Excessive exercise
- Sedentary lifestyle
- Frequent gut infections
- Inflammation in the gut
- Repeat prescriptions of antibiotics
- Stress

- Smoking
- Pregnancy
- Aging
- Gut surgeries

Whether or not most people benefit from supplementing digestive enzymes has not been thoroughly vetted by research, but this is because clinical trials are unlikely to get funded. After all, they don't make pharmaceutical companies a bunch of money. And taking enzyme supplements is very safe and very effective, based on thousands of personal accounts and some verified research.

Did You Know . . . Digestive Enzymes Reduce Gas and Bloating

Research shows that taking digestive enzymes with lipase helps reduce gas, bloating, and feelings of fullness after a large meal.[59] Another study also found that taking the enzyme lipase reduced feelings of fullness after a high-fat meal compared to a placebo.[60] And research shows that digestive enzymes help with IBS symptoms, including bloating, flatulence, diarrhea, and abdominal pain.[61] Research shows that a broad-spectrum enzyme supplement significantly reduces symptoms of bloating and dyspepsia and can help with conditions like mild ulcerative colitis. [62] Even the most prominent critics of dietary supplements acknowledge that lactase enzyme supplements help to improve digestive functions for people who have lactose

[59] Levine M, Koch S, et al. Lipase supplementation before a high-fat meal reduces perceptions of fullness in healthy subjects. *Gut Liver.* 2015 Jul;9(4):464–9.

[60] Suarez F, Levitt M, et al. Pancreatic supplements reduce symptomatic response of healthy subjects to a high fat meal. *Dig Dis Sci.* 1999 Jul;44(7):1317–21.

[61] Ciacci C, Franceschi F, et al. Effect of beta-glucan, inositol and digestive enzymes in GI symptoms of patients with IBS. *Eur Rev Med Pharmacol Sci.* 2011 Jun;15(6):637–43.

[62] Phillips E. Digestive enzymes. *Clinical Education,* 2017. https://www.clinicaleducation.org/news/digestive-enzymes/.

intolerance.[63] However, remember that the more lactose you eat, the more lactase enzymes you need!

Digestive enzymes also have immune-enhancing properties, so they may help with many conditions like colitis or other autoimmune disorders. Additionally, they tend to dampen down inflammatory components of the immune system by helping to break down allergenic compounds before the body absorbs them.

The two most important factors that make up a beneficial digestive enzyme are broad-spectrum enzymes in higher doses. If you eat a complex meal of proteins, fats, and carbohydrates (think your typical roast meat, potatoes, and three veggies), you will want many enzymes to help you break down the food. And if the meal is large, you will need enough enzymes to cover your bases. Each enzyme unit covers a specific amount of food, so the higher the units, ALUs, for example, the more lactose will be digested.

A good digestive enzyme supplement should contain the following:

- Amylase helps digest starch.
- Protease/pancreatin breaks down proteins.
- Lipase breaks down fats.
- Lactase helps digest lactose.
- Glucoamylase is present in saliva and helps to break starch into sugar.
- Sucrase (invertase) breaks glucose into sucrose and fructose.
- Maltase breaks maltose down into sugar.
- Pullulanase breaks down glucan fibers.
- Cellulase breaks down many kinds of fibers.
- Hemicellulase breaks down starches and candida.
- Pectinase breaks down pectin in fruits and vegetables.
- Phytase breaks down phytates (anti-nutrients) in foods.
- Beta-glucanase breaks down beta-glucan fibers.
- Alpha-galactosidase breaks down glycoproteins from beans and legumes

---

[63] Misselwitz B, Butter M, et al. Update on lactose malabsorption and intolerance: pathogenesis, diagnosis and clinical management. *Gut.* 2019 Nov;68(11):2080–91.

(used in Beano®).

- Galactomannase breaks down galactomannan starches.
- Endopeptidases break down proteins into amino acids.

Optional but beneficial enzymes:

- Lysozyme breaks down the cell walls of harmful bacteria and is naturally found in saliva.
- Acid protease is released by the stomach and helps the body digest proteins.
- Alkaline protease digests a wide variety of proteins and is used to reduce allergy symptoms.
- Serratia peptidase helps break down proteins into amino acids; also used for chronic pain, inflammation, and conditions like bronchitis.
- Fructan hydrolase breaks down fructans in high FODMAP foods; great for IBS and SIBO.

The hardest part about digestive enzyme supplements is remembering to take them when you eat. However, I get some relief even if I take them after mealtime. This is because food can be digested over many hours, so all is not lost if you take it late. Many enzyme brands also contain proteases that help break down gluten. You will see on the label that this is listed as DPP-IV activity.

Advisory: Digestive Enzymes Contraindications

Digestive enzymes can help with gluten digestion, but there is no evidence that these enzymes help if you have gluten sensitivity or celiac disease. In fact, I caution against using them for gluten digestion unless you start slowly and test them carefully. By the way, these enzymes don't work for my gluten intolerance.

An enzyme supplement I trust and take is Seeking Health Digestion Intensive, and I also like Amy Myers Complete Enzymes. Both are available directly from the companies online. Another new enzyme supplement for IBS and SIBO that is a good add-on is FODZYME, which contains fructan hydrolase, an enzyme unique to this product that helps people digest foods like wheat, onions, broccoli, and inulin better.

Bile Salts

The gallbladder is the body's reservoir of bile, and if you aren't making enough bile, your body may give subtle or not-so-subtle symptoms. The apparent ones are diarrhea, light-colored stools, foul-smelling gas, or floating fatty stools. Diarrhea makes it so that our body fluids rush out of the body and into the toilet. Bile is one of these precious substances that you lose when you have diarrhea. Long-term diarrhea makes it impossible for the body to keep up with the bile loss. This, in turn, makes it so you can't digest your food well, which further worsens your diarrhea, which means your belly is spiraling out of control. This is called **bile acid malabsorption diarrhea**.

Bile's role is to digest and absorb fats and help remove toxins and heavy metals. Usually, our bodies recycle bile, so around 95 percent of bile is reabsorbed in the small intestine. Our bodies are very effective at conserving their resources, and bile is a precious one. So only under distressing conditions do we run low on it. These conditions include fatty liver, excess alcohol, diarrhea, IBS, pancreatitis, gallstones, gallstone surgery, vitamin D deficiency, menopause, long-term poor diets, and diets low in taurine (vegans).

Other roles for bile in the body include helping to balance the gut microbiome. Bile supplements during weight loss may also reduce the chance of gallstone formation. Bile helps to increase beige fat, which converts white fat into brown fat, which is a good thing because brown fat is more easily metabolized, which improves weight loss.

Acne, eczema, or dry skin can also indicate low bile. It all goes back to a lack of nutrients caused by a lack of absorption or inadequate absorption. Imbalances in your microbiome can also occur because your food is not absorbing well.

Gallbladder removal, or cholecystectomy, is a common type of surgery. Unfortunately, many people continue to have digestive symptoms, such as diarrhea and abdominal pain, afterward. When you remove your gallbladder, you still make bile in the liver, but it trickles into the small intestine. If you eat a big meal, you certainly need more than a trickle of bile to digest your food well. As a result, you can get diarrhea, creating a vicious cycle of low bile.

Ox bile is a prudent supplement to take after gallbladder removal. After all, you probably had your gallbladder removed to feel better, not to digest your foods poorly. Use of bile acids known as TUDCA can reduce diarrhea symptoms and improve dyspepsia as well. A natural way to get bile is to take organ meats that contain gallbladder. They even may help reduce symptoms of food allergies and intolerance. Typical doses are 1-2 grams twice daily at mealtime that include fat.

Bile supplements aren't for everyone, but they certainly can be a lifesaver for people who struggle with the above issues.

Medicinal Mushrooms

All edible mushrooms have medicinal qualities, and the ones particularly known to benefit gut health are Turkey Tail, Reishi, Lion's Mane, and Chaga. As you may recall, your gut is home to most of your immune system, and because of this, mushrooms work their "magic" here. Medicinal mushrooms enhance immune function because they contain many antioxidants and immune-enhancing compounds.

Some mushrooms like Turkey Tail even contain krestin (PSK) and polysaccharide peptide (PSP), which boost immune function and can even be used in helping with cancer treatment. In fact, multiple clinical trials are demonstrating that Turkey Tail mushrooms help reduce cancer complications and are approved for use as part of treatment regimens for cancer in Japan.[64] Because they boost immune function, they can even help fight harmful bacteria like E. coli.

Reishi mushrooms do similar things and also help the body adapt to stress. They are well-known to support immune function via the gut. It even has been clinically shown in research to increase energy levels in people undergoing breast cancer treatment.[65] While Chaga mushrooms may help fight inflammatory bowel diseases by dampening DNA damage due to a reduction in oxidative stress in the body. Chaga mushrooms also help support a healthy liver which enables you to digest foods in return.

All edible mushrooms contain prebiotic fibers which support a healthy gut. Additionally, mushrooms like Lion's Mane help support nerve growth and may reduce symptoms of inflammatory bowel diseases like ulcerative colitis and Crohn's disease by lowering inflammatory compounds such as NFkB and TNFalpha.

Using medicinal mushrooms for gut health is more of a slow and steady game, as consistent daily intake helps more than sporadic use. This is why many people turn to taking these healing mushrooms as supplements. You can find these popular medicinal mushrooms in most health stores and online.

Beetroot

Known primarily for lowering blood pressure, beetroot can improve energy levels and gut health due to its prebiotic fibers. These fibers, known as pectin and pectic-oligosaccharides, help improve the gut microbiome by increasing Bifidobacterium strains of probiotic bacteria. These nutritious vegetables also help increase healthy fats in the gut, called short-chain fatty acids. These

---

[64] Medicinal Mushrooms (PDQ®)–Health Professional Version. National Cancer Institute. https://www.cancer.gov/about-cancer/treatment/cam/hp/mushrooms-pdq.

[65] Zhao H, Zhang Q, et al. Spore powder of Ganoderma lucidum improves cancer-related fatigue in breast cancer patients undergoing endocrine therapy: a pilot clinical trial. *Evid Based Complement Alternat Med.* 2012;2012:809614.

healthy fats feed the gut and maintain a healthy immune system.

Additionally, beets are rich in antioxidants which reduce inflammation that helps protect the gut barrier. And like many antioxidant-rich foods, the benefits of beet powder extend to the liver, which in turn helps gut function. By dampening inflammation compounds like lipopolysaccharides, beetroot is good for dampening the damage of toxins in the liver and in the gut.

If this list of benefits seems appealing to you, but you don't regularly eat beets, beetroot powder or capsules could be the answer. Just keep in mind that, like eating beets, it can turn your stool a pinkish or reddish tint due to its rich antioxidant content of betalains.

Quercetin

Quercetin, a potent antioxidant found in apples and onions, became more widely recognized during the pandemic in 2020. Its uses for health are vastly related to immunity and gut health. Well-known as a natural antihistamine without the bad side effects of conventional antihistamines, this bright yellow antioxidant is also beneficial for the gut.

By promoting gut-healing proteins that seal the gut wall, quercetin holds much promise for those struggling with various gut issues, including **inflammatory bowel disease** and **IBS**. It also helps increase the variety of healthy bacteria in the gut microbiome.

Using quercetin may also help with sluggish bowels because it promotes regularity. It even helps stimulate the production of protective mucin for the gut lining. Some research even indicates that quercetin dampens down the stress response in the body.[66] Often quercetin is combined with vitamin C (see Chapter 6) in supplements; it also is found in combination with nettles or bromelain, both of which are also good for the immune system.

---

[66] Mehta V, Parashar A, et al. Quercetin prevents chronic unpredictable stress induced behavioral dysfunction in mice by alleviating hippocampal oxidative and inflammatory stress. *Physiol Behav.* 2017 Mar 15;171:69–78.

Apple Cider Vinegar (ACV)

The most popular folk remedy for gut health is apple cider vinegar (ACV). Research is admittedly scant, but that doesn't stop the anecdotal evidence of its benefits for indigestion, increasing energy, lowering blood glucose levels, reducing bloating, candida overgrowth, weight loss, and more. Many people say they can stop taking acid reflux medications when they add apple cider vinegar to their diet, and worldwide it has many advocates for its health benefits.

Used as far back as history has been recorded, apple cider vinegar is certainly not bland and without controversy. My only issue with drinking apple cider vinegar is that it may harm tooth enamel over time. This is why taking apple cider vinegar in capsule form makes sense if you want to try it, or you can sip diluted apple cider vinegar with a straw. It is good to have at least two parts water to every part of vinegar and drink it with your main meal. The only way to know if it will improve your digestion is to try taking it. If you feel better, great. If not, you probably shouldn't take it. Otherwise, it is safe to take short-term, but just remember to take it with food.

Chlorella

Chlorella is a single-cell algae natural practitioners use to help cleanse the body. It is also a very nutritious food, so it supports overall health. Rich in prebiotic fibers, chlorella also helps to feed the gut by making the gut's primary fuel source: short-chain fatty acids.

If you recall the benefits of ox bile for people with pale-colored stools and diarrhea, chlorella may help the opposite side of the spectrum; constipation. It also helps to reduce the reabsorption of bile. This, in turn, helps reduce toxins' absorption into the body.

The soil and water are now more contaminated with heavy metals like mercury than ever. And a disrupted microbiome is less likely to be able to clear heavy metals. As a potent detoxifier, research shows that chlorella may even help remove mercury from nerve tissue.[67] Chlorella also benefits the body by decreasing heavy metals in the blood from amalgam or "silver" dental fillings and eliminating it through bowel movements and urine. Chlorella may also help to reduce other heavy metals like cadmium and lead from absorbing into the body. It even helps eliminate perfluorinated compounds and environmental toxins that are toxic to the gut and the whole body.

Chlorella can even improve the quality of life of people with fibromyalgia pain by dampening inflammation and reducing toxins. Research also shows that Chlorella may improve immune function and liver function in hepatitis C and non-alcoholic fatty liver disease. [68]

Taking chlorella isn't always the easiest supplement to take. It is bright green and definitely tastes "healthy." Still, a short-term course for a week or two may help gut function and is a safe thing to try. Some mild side effects can happen, however, such as nausea and increased bowel movements. You can take it with food to avoid these side effects and start with a very low dose. A good starting dose is 3 g per day. Chlorella interacts with warfarin, so talk with your healthcare provider if you are on this medication before taking it.

MCT Oil

MCT oil (medium-chain triglycerides) is a unique type of fat that has a place in gut health regimens for many people. First, it absorbs without the help of the lymphatic system, so it is a quick source of energy for the body. Second, it can reduce candida growth in the gut, which can be a major source of gut issues. Third, it also dampens the growth of harmful bacteria in the gut. Fourth, MCT oil stimulates gut muscle movements, so it can help reduce constipation symptoms. Healthy fats, in general, help to alleviate constipation, but MCT oil shines for this. This means it could be a very

---

[67] Bito T, Okumura E, et al. Potential of chlorella as a dietary supplement to promote human health. *Nutrients.* 2020 Aug 20;12(9):2524.

[68] Moradi M, Behrouj H, et al. Chlorella vulgaris is an effective supplement in counteracting non-alcoholic fatty liver disease-related complications through modulation of dyslipidemia, insulin resistance, and inflammatory pathways. *J Food Biochem.* 2021 Oct;45(10):e13914.

useful tool for helping treat SIBO. Some studies even show it is helpful for inflammatory bowel diseases like ulcerative colitis and Crohn's disease. Not to mention, many people find it very helpful for reducing constipation.

But, you should know that MCT oil should be in the caprylic acid form because if it contains lauric acid, so may negatively affect cholesterol levels. You should also know that because it can act as a laxative, you should try a very small amount at first, such as a teaspoon, and sip it slowly. It is truly powerful in this regard, so the best way to use it is to a small amount of coffee and sip it slowly; otherwise, you may end up with more GI distress.

6

Chapter 6

Essential Vitamins and Minerals for Gut Health

Regarding vitamin and mineral deficiencies, it is important to keep this in perspective: which came first, the chicken or the egg? In other words, did your vitamin and mineral deficiencies cause your gut problems, or did your gut problems cause your vitamin and mineral deficiencies?

The truth is the chicken and the egg came simultaneously. Gut problems can cause vitamin and mineral deficiencies, which can cause gut problems. Let's take the example I gave in Chapter 3 of how refined carbohydrates like sugar or alcohol make your body burn through your vitamin B1 (thiamine) supply. Diabetes, the use of some blood pressure medications, and other issues can cause thiamine deficiency as well. The lack of thiamine, in turn, causes an altered microbiome and may even result in an altered structure of the gut wall due to inflammation. Restoring thiamine in the body helps improve the gut microbiome and helps restore the structural integrity of the gut wall, according to research. [69]

---

[69] Wen K, Zhao M, et al. Thiamine modulates intestinal morphological structure and microbiota under subacute ruminal acidosis induced by a high-concentrate diet in Saanen goats. *Animal.* 2021 Oct;15(10):100370.

Shockingly, vitamin B1 deficiency can look exactly like IBS or SIBO and can even present as constipation. This is because vitamin B1 also helps the body to make acetylcholine, which is a neurotransmitter that is involved in keeping the **vagus nerve** healthy, and therefore is important in gut muscle movements. Lack of vitamin B1 can even reduce stomach acid production, which further causes the gut to become sluggish, leading to bacterial overgrowth. While that sugar load seemed benign at first, you can see how it started a downward spiral of depletion of vitamin B1, which caused your whole body to be out of balance.

The point is that being low in *any* essential nutrient is an absolute detriment to your gut health. You will soon find out how easy it is to be low in any of them and how smart it is to take natural supplements of them.

Case Study: The Path to Health Using a Functional Medicine Perspective

A few things happened in 2018 that changed my life. The first was a local diagnosis of a very rare blood disease. I was told it was probably caused by blood cancer, and I was assigned a local oncologist. Also, I was told to avoid getting cold which curtailed all my winter activities. The oncologist, however, could not find any cancer, and I didn't have any of the symptoms of the blood disease, so eventually, I called Mayo Clinic in Minnesota, and the doctor there, coincidentally doing research on the disease, wanted to see me as quickly as possible. And I didn't have the disease, just the antibodies. This adventure led me to understand an important thing about today's medicine—you must do your own research and care for your health.

Also, early in the year, I caught the H1N1 flu when visiting Australia, and an accompanying bacteria destroyed my microbiome, something I knew nothing about then. After going through a month of every test an MD can do, the persistent abdominal pain had no cause, and I was declared incredibly healthy.

I set out to find the cause and consulted Heidi. I described my history and symptoms, and it didn't take her long to figure out that I had histamine intolerance. As an aside, when I told my very good local doctor, he had no clue what I was talking about. Heidi prescribed a diet and a few supplements. A more in-depth analysis resulted in more supplements to repair the damage done to my microbiome. Since then I haven't looked back. The results have been amazing. Although I probably never will produce the DAO enzyme again that takes care of extra histamine, my microbiome has healed incredibly well, and I can now eat most foods with histamine.

I went from someone who never even took an aspirin to a regular habitue' of health food stores and groceries. I take many supplements every day as they make such a huge difference in how I feel and the strength of my immune system. Quercetin and zinc daily have kept me from catching any viruses. Aside from multivitamins, I also take a B-complex plus B-12, as well as several probiotics daily. *Saccharomyces Boulardii* and drops with *Lactobacillus reuteri* and *Lactobacillus rhamnosus* for my digestion and immune system. Immuse, taken as soon as I get up, helps immensely with my seasonal allergies. When I want to have a glass of wine, I take a DAO supplement 15 minutes before to help with the histamine. And as an aside, I've found that magnesium bound with L-Threonate is wonderful for sleep. And I continue to research and learn. These are exciting times for diet and supplements as so much new research is being done daily. And I have Heidi to thank for all of this.

Vitamins for Vital Health

Vitamins are critical for optimal health and feeling vital. The gut relies on every vitamin in your diet to function at its best, so in the next section, you will learn about these nutrients, who is at risk for having too little, and the research about using these key nutrients as supplements.

Vitamin A for Amazing Gut Healing

As you may recall from Chapter 3, vitamin A is ever-increasingly lacking in our diets, and the gut suffers as a result. This is due, in part, to popular plant-based diets, lack of traditional foods, and our stubborn genes that like for us to get animal-based vitamin A.

To quickly review, vitamin A also protects tissues in the gut from inflammatory compounds and keeps the structure of the gut lining strong. Lack of vitamin A reduces the body's immunity due to imbalances in the gut as well. It regulates over 500 genes, and at least a third of the population doesn't get enough vitamin A based on the **RDI**.[70] The magnitude of the problem is even bigger because the **RDI** is set to only prevent eye issues rather than optimize health.

Signs that you could be low in vitamin A are difficulty seeing at night, bumps on the back of your arms or legs, dry eyes, allergies, insomnia, memory issues, frequent sickness, gut issues, and dry skin. Blood tests, by the way, are not reliable for testing vitamin A deficiency.

To get it out of the way, yes, you can get too much active vitamin A. But higher doses of vitamin A are usually only toxic if your body is also deficient in vitamin D, during pregnancy, or if you have end-stage kidney disease.[71] So, it is important to take vitamin A and vitamin D in tandem. It really also makes sense to get all of the fat-soluble vitamins in adequate amounts for best gut health, including vitamin K2, vitamin E, vitamin A, and vitamin D. More on these shortly.

If you aren't eating organ meats and/or cod liver oil, the best sources of vitamin A, ensure you get vitamin A from a retinol source. Vitamin A is safe to take as retinol. Do not take the beta-carotene form. Beta-carotene likely won't hurt you, but it isn't effective as a vitamin A source for most people.

---

[70] Fulgoni V, Keast D, et al. Foods, fortificants, and supplements: Where do Americans get their nutrients? *J Nutr.* 2011 Oct;141(10):1847–54.

[71] Schoenfeld P. "Vitamin A-Mazing." *The Weston A. Price Foundation*, 2020 May 4. https://www.westonaprice.org/health-topics/vitamin-a-mazing/.

This is because it is poorly absorbed and poorly metabolized, meaning not much of it gets turned into active vitamin A in the body.

Did You Know . . . Higher Doses of Vitamin A Are Safe

Some studies show that doses of 25,000 IU per day of retinol over two months are safe, as done in a study of people with ulcerative colitis who received that dose. [72] Mice, tiny creatures, were given 5000 IU daily, and this dose was safe. Children receiving vitamin A supplements have less diarrhea, reducing their chances of dying in poorer countries. A study done on people with sun-damaged skin received doses of up to 75,000 IU per day for over a year and had no signs of vitamin A toxicity.[73] The internet will scare you away from taking anything more than 10,000 IU per day, so just be aware that this is the dogma out in the world today. But, you should always make sure to take adequate vitamin D along with a good balance of all the other vitamins and minerals to avoid vitamin A toxicity. And high doses aren't always better long term. However, a short-term course over a few weeks of higher doses may help heal the gut more quickly than low doses, in my experience.

Vitamin A may reward you with fewer allergies, improved vision, less sickness, less inflammation, and more. I can't give you an optimal dose as your diet and status are highly unique to you, and there are special concerns like pregnancy, where you should avoid high doses. But, if you take liver or cod liver oil supplements, as reviewed in Chapter 7, and take vitamin D, the balance of nutrients should help you avoid any risk of vitamin A toxicity.

---

[72] Masnadi S, Nikniaz Z, et al. Vitamin A supplementation decreases disease activity index in patients with ulcerative colitis: A randomized controlled clinical trial. *Complement Ther Med.* 2018 Dec;41:215–19.

[73] Alberts D, Ranger-Moore J, et al. Safety and efficacy of dose-intensive oral vitamin A in subjects with sun-damaged skin. *Clin Cancer Res.* 2004 Mar 15;10(6):1875–80.

B Vitamins for Balanced Gut

We have already reviewed the impact of vitamin B1 and how it can easily get out of balance in the body. It is just as easy to fall short in all the other B vitamins because we don't have a lot of storage for these water-soluble vitamins.

The B vitamins and best forms are:

· Vitamin B1 thiamine
· Vitamin B2 riboflavin
· Vitamin B3 niacin (niacinamide, nicotinic acid)
· Vitamin B5 pantothenic acid
· Vitamin B6 pyridoxine (best supplemented as pyridoxal-5-phosphate)
· Vitamin B7 biotin
· Vitamin B9 folate (do not choose folic acid; choose 5-MTHF, folinic acid, or methylfolate)
· Vitamin B12 cobalamin (choose methylcobalamin or adenosylcobalamin; do not choose cyanocobalamin)

Stress, sugar, medications, processed foods, an altered microbiome, gut conditions like IBS and SIBO, and inflammation can make you low in many B vitamins. For this reason, it makes sense to combine them in either a natural B-complex supplement or a broad-spectrum multivitamin with minerals.

Sounds easy, right?

Not really. This is because many brands today pose as natural and are not. Here is why you need to seek out natural B vitamins instead of synthetic forms.

Did You Know . . . Your Genes Affect Vitamin B Absorption

In 1943, scientists learned how to make artificial folate as folic acid. Although very close structurally to folate, folic acid has a key difference that requires a specific gene variant in your body to convert it to the active form. Folic acid also requires a conversion in your gut to become active. As it turns out, up to half of people have a variant in this gene,[74] so folic acid gets "jammed up" in the body. This gene variant is called MTHFR polymorphism.

It's easier to tell you the brands of vitamins that you can trust than to tell you what to avoid because there are so many to avoid.

Vitamin C for Critical Gut Immunity

As you may recall from Chapter 3, vitamin C deficiency is pretty common due to inflammation, being overweight, stress, and common medications like antacids. Taking vitamin C is definitely more straightforward than some other nutrients because it would be difficult to take too much. Higher doses can have some pretty amazing benefits for dampening down symptoms of inflammation and allergies too. For example, during allergy season, taking 1 g (1000 mg) of vitamin C multiple times a day can be a really simple trick to reduce symptoms without taking allergy drugs with harmful long-term side effects.

When it comes to gut health, vitamin C helps many things. For example, high doses of vitamin C at 1000 mg daily improved the gut microbiome diversity in healthy people.[75] Vitamin C also helps to reduce the absorption of toxins into the bloodstream as well by helping to strengthen the gut barrier. And it goes without saying that vitamin C is critical for a healthy immune response housed in the gut. And the combination of vitamin C and probiotics likely have synergistic effects. One study showed that both helped to decrease days of upper respiratory tract infections by twenty-one days over six months compared to no probiotics or vitamin C in children.[76] Taking extra vitamin C

---

[74] Anderson S, Panka J, et al. Anxiety and methylenetetrahydrofolate reductase mutation treated with s-adenosyl methionine and methylated B vitamins. *Integr Med (Encinitas).* 2016 Apr;15(2):48–52.

[75] Otten A, Bourgonje A, et al. Vitamin C supplementation in healthy individuals leads to shifts of bacterial populations in the gut-a pilot study. *Antioxidants (Basel).* 2021 Aug 12;10(8):1278.

[76] Garaiova I, Muchová J, et al. Probiotics and vitamin C for the prevention of respiratory tract infections in children attending preschool: a randomized controlled pilot study. *Eur J Clin Nutr.* 2015 Mar;69(3):373–9.

can also be a quick and safe trick to help alleviate constipation.

You can get many forms of vitamin C, such as liposomal, for optimal absorption. I like combining liposomal vitamin C and vitamin C from acerola or rose hips. The liposomal is absorbed more readily into the bloodstream, but the acerola and rose hips forms both have quick actions in the gut. Interestingly, the ester form of vitamin C is related to a reduced risk of urinary oxalate levels, potentially reducing the risk of kidney stones.[77]

The dogma stands that you can only absorb a small amount of vitamin C at a time. Even if so, it doesn't matter because your gut can use the extra to dampen histamines and inflammation. And the risk of kidney stones and vitamin C remains fairly unsubstantiated in research: some studies show less risk of kidney stones, and some show more risk.[78] It's probably just a lot of white noise, as is often the case in population studies. Using a quick risk-benefit analysis shows that vitamin C has little to no risk with a high chance of benefit for many.[79]

Vitamin D for Dynamic Gut Health

Vitamin D supplements are powerful for gut health. They help to reduce the severity of daunting conditions like inflammatory bowel diseases, including ulcerative colitis and Crohn's disease. In fact, twelve studies show that this is the case, and high doses of vitamin D supplements worked better than low doses.[80] Four studies found the same to be true in people who suffer from

[77] Otten A, Bourgonje A, et al. Vitamin C supplementation in healthy individuals leads to shifts of bacterial populations in the gut-a pilot study. *Antioxidants (Basel)*. 2021 Aug 12;10(8):1278.

[78] Ferraro P, Curhan G, et al. Total, dietary, and supplemental vitamin C intake and risk of incident kidney stones. *Am J Kidney Dis*. 2016 Mar;67(3):400–7.

[79] Li J, Chen N, et al. Efficacy of vitamin D in treatment of inflammatory bowel disease: A meta-analysis. *Medicine (Baltimore)*. 2018 Nov;97(46):e12662.

[80] Xu K, Peng R, et al. Vitamin C intake and multiple health outcomes: an umbrella review of systematic reviews and meta-analyses. *Int J Food Sci Nutr*. 2022 Aug;73(5):588–99.

IBS. [81] IBS and SIBO are also tightly related, so vitamin D is helpful for SIBO too. Vitamin D is great at dampening inflammation and helping to balance out the immune system in so many ways.

Probiotic supplements aren't the only players that can improve the gut microbiome; it turns out that vitamin D has a positive role on the healthy bacteria that reside in the gut by increasing bacterial diversity. It even plays a role in pancreas and gallbladder health, and too little vitamin D in the body can create inflammation in these tissues.

Vitamin D is an important factor in every aspect of health because it acts as a hormone, so there isn't a cell in your body that doesn't suffer if you are low in vitamin D, especially your gut cells.

Did You Know . . . It Is Vital to Check Your Vitamin D Levels

It is critical to check your blood levels, as it is one nutrient with accurate blood levels. The media doesn't give vitamin D the generous respect that it deserves. And remember the Flexner report from Chapter 4? Doctors were silenced about natural treatments starting in the early 1900s, so their breadth of knowledge on vitamin D can be sadly narrow. So you have to be your own best advocate when it comes to vitamin D by getting your blood levels checked at least twice a year. If your healthcare provider doesn't check your levels, find a new provider. Or you can get online vitamin D test kits that are as accurate or more accurate than the ones that your doctor can provide. It really is that important. Disease risk plummets at the blood level of 50 ng/ml, and your well-being can rise. The test you are looking for is called 25-hydroxyvitamin D.

Vitamin D protects your gut in so many dynamic ways. It helps keep autoimmune conditions in check when in balance with a good diet, helps heart function, keeps the gut from excessive inflammation, supports brain

---

[81] Chong RIH, Yaow CYL, Loh CYL, Teoh SE, Masuda Y, Ng WK, Lim YL, Ng QX. Vitamin D supplementation for irritable bowel syndrome: A systematic review and meta-analysis. J Gastroenterol Hepatol. 2022 Jun;37(6):993-1003..

health via the gut-brain axis, and more. But, like most nutrients, you must balance them with many other nutrients, especially vitamin A, vitamin K2, magnesium, biotin, and more. Our bodies are one big symphony of nutrients.

Vitamin D dosing can be a little tricky. One vitamin D IU listed on vitamin labels equals 0.025 mg of vitamin D. This is super tiny, and you can't see it with the naked eye. The units are deceptive. For example, 5000 IU of vitamin D3 is 125 mg or about a tenth of a milligram. It would fit on the tip of a pencil eraser.

Sun exposure that turns your skin a different shade gives you about 25,000 IU of vitamin D but does come with the risk of sun damage. In contrast, a glass of milk gives you only 100 IU of vitamin D, leaving you very deficient. The **RDI** leaves most people deficient in vitamin D, but again, **RDIs** are not established to make you healthy; they are established to keep you from dying from deficiency.

People are almost all deficient or suboptimal in vitamin D unless they work outside in the sun. When I worked in a hospital, we measured over 400 hospital employees' blood, and 95 percent had insufficient levels. Those that weren't low were likely supplementing vitamin D.

This means that basically, everyone needs to take supplemental vitamin D, but the amount you need is highly dependent on your genetics. Most people need at least 2000 IU per day and often more. One final point on this topic; over-the-counter vitamin D3 is natural, safe, and more effective than the prescription variety, vitamin D2.

If you are worried about toxicity, yes, vitamin D can reach toxic levels, but it is exceedingly rare and always reversible. To be sure, it is always best to check both serum calcium and 25-hydroxyvitamin D levels when you are supplementing vitamin D. The true marker of toxicity of vitamin D is not the vitamin D blood level but elevated serum calcium. For an in-depth review of vitamin D and its range of safety, visit Painscience.com.

Vitamin E: The Knowns and Unknowns

You might be starting to think that all nutrients affect the gut microbiome, and you would be right—even vitamin E. This isn't too surprising, either, because vitamin E is a potent antioxidant, and they help to regulate the gut microbiome. Vitamin E helps to protect the gut and make the intestinal cells function better. However, beyond this, little is known about the full role that vitamin E has in protecting the gut. So, until we know more, it is important to balance it in the diet.

Foods rich in vitamin E include spices like annatto, paprika, chilis, nuts, and seeds, especially hulled pumpkin seeds, poppy seeds, walnuts, sunflower seeds, and peanuts. These foods should be soaked, sprouted, and fermented for the best gut health. You can get some vitamin E in foods like wheat germ and amaranth, but these have gut-triggering issues for many, so I like to provide that warning and recommend sticking to spices, nuts, and seeds.

Like most nutrients, the story can get complicated because of the symphony of the actions of vitamin E and other nutrients. Vitamin E isn't one vitamin, but eight, as it turns out. There are four types of vitamin E in the category of tocopherols and four types of vitamin E in the category of tocotrienols. All eight types have overlapping bodily functions, such as protecting them from free radicals and oxidative stress. They also all have slightly varying functions, making them unique and important.

This is one reason you should avoid synthetic vitamin E, which comes in one form called dl-alpha tocopherol that doesn't function as well as natural varieties. Vitamin E in natural forms is quite safe at moderate doses in adults from supplements and from foods. It is important to know that up to now, no optimal amount of vitamin E has been established yet. But, if you go to the store and pick up the most common and inexpensive vitamin E, it is likely to be an artificial variety of alpha-tocopherol called dl-alpha-tocopherol. So always choose the natural varieties, even if they are more expensive.

Did You Know . . . Not to Waste Your Money on Synthetic Supplements

Synthetic vitamin E is similar to natural vitamin E but not similar enough. A research study found that synthetic vitamin E is also lost in the urine three times faster than natural vitamin E. [82] Vitamin E levels may increase more in our cells with natural vitamin E than synthetic vitamin E, so natural vitamin E is much more effective. This is because synthetic vitamin E displaces a critically important type of vitamin E called gamma-tocopherol, which may increase cancer risk.[83] Synthetic vitamin E is found in packaged foods like breakfast cereals, standard multivitamins, and even eye vitamins heavily marketed to people, sadly. It is in supplement drinks in the hospital and for people who need to gain weight. It is cheap but not benign. Synthetic vitamin E may raise all kinds of havoc in the body, especially at high doses of over 400 IU. It is linked to a significantly increased risk of strokes, pneumonia, skin cancer, liver damage, and more. For all of these reasons, you should avoid synthetic vitamin E.

Vitamin K2: The Superior Vitamin K

Vitamin K2 governs all vitamin K actions in the body, and research shows it is an important nutrient for digestive tract health.[84] [85]It helps to reduce

[82] Traber M, Elsner A, et al. Synthetic as compared with natural vitamin E is preferentially excreted as alpha-CEHC in human urine: studies using deuterated alpha-tocopheryl acetates. *FEBS Lett.* 1998 Oct 16;437(1–2):145–8.

[83] Xin J, Jiang X, et al. Association between circulating vitamin E and ten common cancers: evidence from large-scale Mendelian randomization analysis and a longitudinal cohort study. *BMC Med* 20:168 (2022).

[84] Sogabe N, Maruyama R, et al. Enhancement effects of vitamin K1 (phylloquinone) or vitamin K2 (menaquinone-4) on intestinal alkaline phosphatase activity in rats. *J Nutr Sci Vitaminol (Tokyo).* 2007 Jun;53(3):219–24.

[85] Sultana H, Watanabe K, et al. Effects of vitamin K_2 on the expression of genes involved in bile acid synthesis and glucose homeostasis in mice with humanized PXR. *Nutrients.* 2018 Jul 27;10(8):982.

inflammation in the gut, balance gut-derived immunity, strengthen the gut lining by reducing leaky gut, and make digestive enzymes. Some research even shows that it may reduce the risk of digestive cancers like colon cancer and liver cancer. [86]

If you currently suffer from a gut issue, you are more likely to lose vitamin K2 and become deficient. Medications also can rob you of vitamin K, such as cholesterol-lowering drugs, antibiotics, laxatives, and warfarin.

The list of foods that are rich in vitamin K2 is short, and it includes natto, goose liver, grass-fed cheeses, egg yolks, grass-fed butter, beef liver, and chicken liver. Natto contains much more vitamin K2 than any of these foods at around 1000 mcg per serving compared to less than 100 mcg for the rest of the foods on the list.

Most people are deficient in vitamin K2 because it is so rare in foods. Some scientists argue that it can be made in the gut, but this would be under ideal microbial conditions. And if you are reading this book, I'm sure you may not fit into this category. No one knows if they have an ideal microbiome because what is ideal for you might be entirely different for the next person. Scientists know that most healthy people still have low levels of vitamin K2 in their blood.

Vitamin K2 may play a role in keeping the gut lining intact. This is because it helps to increase a compound called alkaline phosphatase activity in the epithelial lining. This increase in alkaline phosphatase helps to reduce inflammation in the gut and reduces toxins known as lipopolysaccharides. Another way that vitamin K2 may help protect the gut is by reducing leaky gut. It effectively helps seal the gut and prevents invasion from unwanted toxins and microbes. It does this by increasing a compound called pregnane X receptor which may prevent harmful bacteria from entering the bloodstream. Vitamin K2 may also be involved in making digestive enzymes in the pancreas and regulating bile in the liver. The first line of evidence for this argument is that the pancreas contains a lot of vitamin K2. These enzymes made by

---

[86] Xv F, Chen J, et al. Research progress on the anticancer effects of vitamin K2. *Oncol Lett.* 2018 Jun;15(6):8926–34.

the pancreas are required to help you digest your foods properly. Bile helps to absorb fats and vitamins. While we don't know the exact role vitamin K2 plays in bile production, it does influence the genes that control it.

Did You Know . . . Vitamin K2 Protects Health in Several Ways

Vitamin K2 plays a role in both innate and adaptive immune function. Research shows that vitamin K2 helps to modulate T-cell proliferation, which may allow for a more balanced immune response. Using vitamin K2 in kidney transplant patients helped to increase IL-4 levels from peripheral blood mononuclear cells (PBMCs). [87] Increasing IL-4 may help protect bone tissues and reduce an overactive immune response. A few research papers show that taking vitamin K2 may not only reduce cancer risk but also may help enhance cancer treatment.[88]

When your gut isn't absorbing foods well due to digestive conditions like ulcerative colitis, Crohn's disease, or celiac disease, your body can't absorb vitamin K well either. Inflammatory bowel diseases also make it so your microbiome isn't as robust as it could be, making any chances that your body will make vitamin K2 very low. In other words, if you struggle with digestive issues, you should focus on eating vitamin K2-rich foods and consider adding supplements. Most multivitamin supplements contain a paltry amount of vitamin K2, so it makes sense to buy vitamin K2 as menaquinone. The most well-tested vitamin K2 supplement is the patented MenaQ7®. You can find this kind of vitamin K2 in combination with vitamin D because they both tend to be scant in multivitamin supplements. Just make sure to check with your healthcare provider before taking vitamin K2 if you are on warfarin.

---

[87] Kusano J, Tanaka S, et al. Vitamin K1 and Vitamin K2 immunopharmacological effects on the peripheral lymphocytes of healthy subjects and dialysis patients, as estimated by the lymphocyte immunosuppressant sensitivity test. *J Clin Pharm Ther.* 2018 Dec;43(6):895–902.

[88] Xv F, Chen J, et al. Research progress on the anticancer effects of vitamin K2. *Oncol Lett.* 2018 Jun;15(6):8926–34.

Magnificent Minerals

The gut relies on minerals for many aspects of repairing and maintaining healthy gut cells. But, like vitamins, many types of minerals can be deficient in the diet of just about anyone due to modern farming practices and processed foods. Learn about the benefits of each mineral and if and when you should consider supplementing these critical nutrients.

Magnesium for Maintenance and Regulation

Magnesium has seemingly endless benefits for the body. It is required for no less than 300 enzymatic reactions in the body. Most of us don't get enough magnesium due to soil depletion.

Specifically, in the gut, magnesium helps to prevent constipation, binds unwanted compounds like oxalates, relaxes the gut muscles, and helps to heal a leaky gut. Magnesium naturally helps to create a balanced microbiome as well. Sadly, deficiency of magnesium contributes to inflammation in the gut as well.

Magnesium deficiency is very common, and supplements can help reduce gut issues and pain in the body. Not only is magnesium involved in vitamin D metabolism, but your vitamin D stores may also drop if you don't have enough magnesium in your system. And if you don't eat green vegetables, nuts, and seeds daily, you run an extra high risk of magnesium deficiency. Also, like many nutrients, common medications may rob you of magnesium.

Generally, magnesium supplements between 200–400 mg are safe for most adults. You should always choose a highly absorbable kind of magnesium to avoid side effects and for maximal benefit. Personally, I prefer to get magnesium in a powder, but you can also choose a magnesium supplement in capsule or gelcap form. I like magnesium glycinate for its added gut benefits with its glycinate content if you are looking for gut healing.

Many people also find a powder form of magnesium carbonate helpful as it helps constipation and benefits sleep. Research shows that the magnesium oxide form of magnesium supplements is particularly beneficial for ongoing constipation.[89] But regardless of the type chosen, it is always better absorbed in a gelcap, capsule, liquid, or powder form, as tablet forms are poorly absorbed.

Calcium for Healthy Bacteria

Diets high in calcium are generally related to an improved gut microbiome. Specifically, increased calcium intake is related to abundant *Lactobacillus* bacteria in the gut. Calcium appears to have an effect on the gut similar to prebiotics in that it stimulates the growth of healthy bacteria. Beyond that, however, little is known about the interplay of calcium as a nutrient and gut health. For this reason, it makes sense to eat calcium-rich foods, but supplements aren't necessary beyond that unless indicated by your healthcare practitioner.

Calcium-rich foods that can also be good for the gut are canned sardines and salmon, plain yogurt (unsweetened), kefir, aged cheeses, cooked leafy greens, broccoli, sprouted almonds, and soaked and sprouted seeds like chia. I don't recommend calcium-fortified foods because these foods are usually highly processed and unhealthy for the gut.

Iron: Balance is Key

Iron deficiency is a newly recognized cause of gut microbiome imbalances. For example, low iron levels may decrease the type of bacteria that make healthy gut compounds like butyrate. On the other hand, iron excess doesn't seem to harm the gut microbiome.

An extremely fascinating aspect of gut health is that probiotic supplements can enhance the absorption of iron in people who have iron deficiency. For example, a type of probiotic called *Lactobacillus plantarum* helps prevent

---

[89] Mori S, Tomita T, Fujimura K, Asano H, Ogawa T, Yamasaki T, Kondo T, Kono T, Tozawa K, Oshima T, Fukui H, Kimura T, Watari J, Miwa H. A Randomized Double-blind Placebo-controlled Trial on the Effect of Magnesium Oxide in Patients With Chronic Constipation. J Neurogastroenterol Motil. 2019 Oct 30;25(4):563-575.

iron deficiency. However, that's not the end of the story. If you have an inflammatory bowel disease like ulcerative colitis, your gut wall is too inflamed, and it can't absorb the iron well. This extra iron left in the gut can wreak havoc and is thought to increase the risk of colon cancer. And genetic conditions like iron overload can cause similar risks to the gut if you eat too much iron for your genes.

The answer to iron deficiency in inflammatory bowel diseases may also be the addition of probiotics, but research needs to prove this. A good anti-inflammatory diet geared towards autoimmune conditions should also help too.

Remember that iron deficiency very common worldwide, especially in women and children. So, the concern of too much iron is typically limited to men with genetically predisposed iron overload and older women who are menopausal. You will often know if you have this condition if your blood levels of hemoglobin are too high. People with this condition often donate blood to help reduce their health risks.

For everyone else with iron deficiency, I recommend getting iron from organ meats like grass-fed beef liver, heart, and spleen. If you don't eat these foods, you can supplement them, as reviewed in Chapter 7. Iron supplements are also widely used, and iron bisglycinate is often easiest on the stomach.

Sodium: Necessary Trace Minerals

Sodium, better known as salt, despite its bad name, is an essential nutrient that functions as an electrolyte in your gut and throughout your whole body. If you eat a more ancestral diet, you will not have to worry about too much salt. Using a pinch of Himalayan salt now and then provides not only sodium but necessary trace minerals too.

In fact, some people with gut disorders run too low in sodium, such as chronic diarrhea. If you sweat a lot or use sauna/heat therapies to induce sweating, the salt in your diet can be very liberal. Most studies looking at the negative effects of too low sodium on the gut are quite old, but they found that a relative lack of salt can cause gut muscle movements to be impaired.[90]

If you are an athlete or sweat a lot, you may need to replace electrolytes, including sodium. A good electrolyte replacement can be very beneficial for **intermittent fasting**, which is a healthy practice for the gut and improves the **migrating motor complex** function.

Still, it is very possible to get too much salt, especially if you eat processed foods often. This can potentially impair the gut microbiome's health. Just say no to processed foods for the most part.

Potassium for Gut Integrity

Only around half of Americans eat enough potassium in a day, and deficiency is linked to a leaky gut and thereby allowing unwanted bacteria to enter the bloodstream.

Potassium-rich foods are easy to add to the diet. They include pumpkin, sweet potatoes, yogurt, most root vegetables, meats, fish, prunes, papaya, pineapple, cooked leafy greens, oranges, kiwis, squash, avocados, mushrooms, dark chocolate, tomatoes, bananas, melons, dried fruits, and more. Hence supplementing potassium usually doesn't make much sense because it is bulky and cumbersome to take. Still, you can get several electrolyte drinks; see page 304 for my recommended brands.

Zinc: The Warm Blanket Mineral

As far as minerals go, zinc is the most healing mineral to add if you have many gut conditions. Zinc helps to heal gut cells and increase the protection of the gut mucosal lining. This is especially true if you use a form of zinc called zinc carnosine. Using zinc carnosine is particularly healing in the case of stomach ulcers, and research shows that it can work even better than conventional

---

[90] Sahay M, Sahay R. Hyponatremia: A practical approach. *Indian J Endocrinol Metab.* 2014 Nov;18(6):760–71.

drug treatment for this condition. [91] It is even helpful in dampening inflammation and symptoms of people struggling with ulcerative colitis. Zinc even helps improve the microbiome, as new research is indicating.[92]

Zinc has established roles in its benefits on innate immune function and by dampening inflammation. But, zinc deficiency can be hard to identify because blood tests aren't particularly accurate as zinc is stored in muscle tissue and organs, not the blood. Deficiency can contribute to muscle pains and cramps in certain people. While zinc deficiency is less common than vitamin D or magnesium deficiency, the following groups risk being low in zinc: vegetarians and vegans, older adults, people taking prescription medications, people who drink alcohol, people with diabetes, athletes, or people eating nutrient-poor diets.

A question to ask yourself about your diet related to zinc: Does your diet contain mostly pasta, grains, legumes, beans, and rice? While these foods do have some zinc, they are bound and hard to digest the zinc due to antinutrients. You can find zinc carnosine at health food stores, naturopath dispensaries, or on Fullscript.

Advisory: Don't Overdo the Zinc

If you take zinc carnosine, stick to doses used in research: 75–150 mg of zinc carnosine per day for around eight weeks. This provides 17–35 mg of elemental zinc. Just remember to take it with food because, like most minerals, it absorbs better, and you will feel better too. Most multivitamins with minerals contain around 15–20 mg of zinc per serving. If you do take a multivitamin with minerals as well, it still should be fine in the short term of eight weeks to take zinc carnosine and not get too much. If you take zinc carnosine for longer, it could interfere with your body's storage of copper.

---

[91] Efthymakis K, Neri M. The role of Zinc L-Carnosine in the prevention and treatment of gastrointestinal mucosal disease in humans: a review. *Clin Res Hepatol Gastroenterol.* 2022 Aug–Sep;46(7):101954.

[92] Zackular J, Moore J, et al. Dietary zinc alters the microbiota and decreases resistance to Clostridium difficile infection. *Nat Med.* 2016 Nov;22(11):1330–34.

Trace minerals

Regarding most trace minerals, there is only a trace amount of research about how they affect our health. The exceptions are selenium, iodine, chromium, boron, copper, and molybdenum. Here is an overview of what is known and not known about these minerals and gut health in this section.

Selenium

As a potent antioxidant, selenium is important in immune and gut health. Low selenium levels alter the gut microbiome in a way that increases the risk of gut issues like inflammatory bowel diseases. Selenium works in tandem with iodine to help keep the thyroid healthy. The typical pitfalls of westernized diets, lifestyles, and medications can make you low in selenium.

The soil content of selenium varies wildly from place to place, so some people end up with too little. Eating Brazil nuts and seafood is a great way to get a natural source of selenium if you eat them regularly. But even Brazil nuts vary greatly in their selenium content due to soil conditions. To get enough selenium, pick a broad-spectrum multivitamin with minerals with around 50–100 mcg of selenium as selenomethionine.

Iodine

As mentioned previously, it is ideal to aim for plenty of selenium and iodine simultaneously. Both protect the body against toxins like excess chlorine, fluorine, and bromine. Iodine-rich foods also almost always happen to be rich in selenium, such as shellfish and seafood. If you don't eat shellfish or seafood regularly, you should make sure your multivitamin with minerals contains iodine in it to help maintain a healthy thyroid. But little is known about the direct effects of iodine on the gut.

Chromium

Chromium is an interesting mineral because it is both an essential nutrient but also falls in the category of heavy metals. Because of this, a narrower window of safety exists for this essential nutrient. Some early research shows that chromium helps maintain healthy gut bacteria by increasing good bacteria such as *Lactobacillus*. [93] Interestingly, a healthy microbiome also protects the body from excess chromium.

This mineral is fairly widespread in whole foods, such as meats, fruits, and vegetables, but is stripped away if foods are processed. If you supplement chromium, up to 1000 mcg per day appears to be safe. Most high-quality multivitamins with minerals listed above contain a moderate amount of chromium.

Boron

Boron is a little-discussed but fascinating trace mineral because it enhances the effectiveness of other nutrients like magnesium and vitamin D in the body. On its own, it acts to help dampen inflammation, helps protect the body from pesticides and toxins, and may even reduce the risk of cancer. Typically, you can find boron in fruits and vegetables as well as dairy and coffee. Many parts of the world have soils that are low in boron, including most of the United States, so foods that contain boron vary tremendously.

Low doses of boron from supplements may protect the gut, but high doses may actually harm the gut. Luckily, most foods and common supplements, such as the ones listed in the B-vitamins section of this chapter (see page 84), don't contain high doses of boron, only low or moderate doses.

---

[93] Wang G, Li X, et al. Effects of dietary chromium picolinate on gut microbiota, gastrointestinal peptides, glucose homeostasis, and performance of heat-stressed broilers. *Animals* (Basel). 2022 Mar 27;12(7):844.

Molybdenum

Molybdenum is a mineral that remains a bit of a mystery overall. However, some research shows that this mineral helps to reduce the harmful effects of candida overgrowth in the gut. [94] It may also reduce the chances that you have a sulfite sensitivity because it helps convert sulfite to sulfate. Interestingly, it also plays a role in detoxifying alcohol and drugs in the liver.

Like boron, molybdenum content in soils varies a lot, so the content of your food does as well. Typically, you can find molybdenum in most fruits, nuts, beef liver, vegetables, and dairy. Beans also contain molybdenum, but beans are notoriously problematic for people with gut issues. It is also poorly absorbed from beans because of its phytic acid content.

As with other trace minerals, trace amounts are often enough for health, but little research has been done to establish ideal molybdenum intake at this point in time.

Copper

Copper is a double-edged sword when it comes to health. Too little can result in anemia and overgrowth of bacteria, while too much can cause gut toxicity with symptoms like diarrhea, abdominal pain, nausea, and vomiting. Excess copper almost always occurs because people either use copper pipes for their water supply or drink/cook with copper cooking utensils. Copper deficiency can occur in people with inflammatory bowel conditions and poor absorption.

Eating copper-rich foods seems to be enough for health because these foods also tend to be rich in zinc, which helps to balance out copper in the body. Copper-rich foods include beef liver, nuts, seeds, shellfish, and chocolate.

---

[94] Zackular J, Moore J, et al. Dietary zinc alters the microbiota and decreases resistance to Clostridium difficile infection. *Nat Med.* 2016 Nov;22(11):1330–34.

7

Chapter 7

Culinary Herbs and Spices for Gut Healing

If there is an area of untapped health benefits in conventional medicine, it is herbs and spices. My life has forever been changed for the better by various herbs, and I would shout it from the rooftop if I could. Herbs and spices for digestion are unsung heroes, so I'm excited to share this chapter with you. I actually want to write an entire book about how using herbs, with the help of my naturopath, has helped my hormonal issues to go away as well. But I digress.

This chapter will introduce some herbs and spices that help digestive function. Each of the following chapters will delve into when and how to use these herbs for various conditions like IBS, constipation, diarrhea, and more.

A Bit of Herbal History

Before we continue, I would like to share some of the little-known history of herbal medicine. As I shared in Chapter 4, the Flexner Report meant that plant medicine became a lost art. The science of plant medicine, even conducted today, remains largely neglected because the funneling and dissemination of resources in healthcare today are almost exclusively dedicated to pharmaceuticals. It doesn't have to be this way, as herbs are famous for their entourage effects which means each herb has not one use but many. A single herb can contain over 200 beneficial compounds, so it isn't just an entourage; it is synergism that helps your body. Prescription medications, while sometimes necessary, just can't compete with herbs' complex benefits.

You always check with your healthcare provider before taking herbal supplements. Still, generally, herbs and spices are usually safe add-ins to your health routine and have thousands of years of recorded safety. And for sure, if you are allergic or sensitive to any of them, please don't use them.

A–Z Herbs

Generally speaking, the following herbal remedies (listed alphabetically) are very safe when consumed in tea form or in food and beverage recipes. When taking herbs as supplements, you should look for herbs with standardized extracts and herbal supplements that have Good Manufacturing Practices (GMP) certification when possible. This is usually listed on the label.

Certain brands meet rigorous quality criteria and are available to healthcare practitioners through Fullscript. In other words, you are more likely to get what you intend to buy if you use a reputable source like this compared to other retailers. For example, some supplement sellers market fake products, which you definitely don't want.

Typically, a safe dose of herbs and spices will be listed on the label, but for certain conditions, you may need to take more or less. Obviously, if you grow your own herbs or buy them fresh or dried, there is no label, so you should look for herbs with a fragrant smell characteristic of each herb. A good practice is to open up your first capsule and smell it-your senses are your first guide. In other words, if it walks like a duck, it is a duck.

Most herbs and spices work better and will settle on your stomach better if you eat them with food, especially a meal with healthy fat. And last but not least, it's important to remember that what is good for one person is not always good for the next. We can be unique in our response to spices and herbs, but this is true of conventional medications.

Aloe Vera

This easy-to-grow plant has some interesting benefits for your gut. First, it helps to increase the muscle movements of the intestines. Second, it increases the water content of the colon. And finally, it also stimulates the production of mucus in the gut. Doing these three things is helpful for constipation and constipation-predominant types of IBS. Containing around 200 active compounds, aloe has many external and internal uses.

In fact, a review of three clinical trials concluded that aloe vera is a safe and beneficial treatment for IBS.[95] [96] If you want aloe vera supplements, I suggest finding a reputable source like Fullscript, which carries pharmaceutical-grade supplements.

Bay Leaves

While bay leaves may not be on your radar as helpful for digestion, they certainly are.[97] They are super versatile to use in cooking and have gas-reducing properties. Rich in antioxidants, they may help protect the GI tract from toxins as well.

Adding bay leaves to the pot when cooking beans helps soften them for easier digestion, but make sure to properly soak and ferment them first. Also, discard the leaves after cooking since they are indigestible. You can add bay

---

[95] Hong S, Chun J, et al. Aloe vera Is effective and safe in short-term treatment of irritable bowel syndrome: a systematic review and meta-analysis. *J Neurogastroenterol Motil.* 2018 Oct 1;24(4):528-535.

[96] Foster M, Hunter D, et al. Evaluation of the nutritional and metabolic effects of aloe vera. In: Benzie IFF, Wachtel-Galor S, editors. *Herbal Medicine: Biomolecular and Clinical Aspects.* 2nd edition. Boca Raton (FL): CRC Press/Taylor & Francis; 2011. Chapter 3. Available from: https://www.ncbi.nlm.nih.gov/books/NBK92765/

[97] Speroni E, Cervellati R, et al. Gastroprotective effect and antioxidant properties of different Laurus nobilis L. leaf extracts. *J Med Food.* 2011 May;14(5):499-504.

leaves to just about any dish you can think of because their mild flavor offers a subtle flavor to foods. A rule of thumb is to add three to six leaves per dish.

Cannabis

Although cannabis remains hotly debated and legal only for 75 percent of people in the United States, many people who struggle with chronic abdominal pain find relief from this medicinal herb. Cannabis has undisputed anti-inflammatory properties and helps with many chronic pain conditions.

Did You Know . . . Many Clinical Studies Show the Benefits of Cannabis Use

Clinical studies show that cannabis may help reduce acid reflux and the severity of inflammatory bowel diseases by dampening inflammation in the stomach while reducing abdominal pain naturally.[98] In fact, fifty-one studies, mostly animal studies, show a benefit to using cannabis with numerous gut issues. [99] In people with autoimmune-related gut conditions, 45 percent reach remission with cannabis use, reducing cancer risk.[100] Remember that these studies aren't classically controlled double-blind, so more research is needed. While I could keeping saying that more research is needed, it is also a therapy that has been used for thousands of years with a high safety track record for most.

Alternatively, you can purchase CBD but buy a full spectrum oil from a company you know and trust. There are a lot of fairly questionable CBD products on the market. The best way to know what you are getting is to get

[98] Naftali T, Bar-Lev Schleider L, et al. Cannabis induces a clinical response in patients with Crohn's disease: a prospective placebo-controlled study. *Clin Gastroenterol Hepatol.* 2013 Oct;11(10):1276–80.e1.

[99] Couch D, Maudslay H, et al. The Use of Cannabinoids in Colitis: A Systematic Review and Meta-Analysis. *Inflamm Bowel Dis.* 2018 Mar 19;24(4):680–97.

[100] Ravikoff Allegretti J, et al. Marijuana use patterns among patients with inflammatory bowel disease. *Inflamm Bowel Dis.* 2013 Dec;19(13):2809–14.

cannabis flower or high-CBD cannabis in flower form or RSO oil.

Whatever your choice, starting at a very low dose is your best bet. I highly recommend listening to the Cannabis Health Radio podcast with Cory Yelland for tips on medically using cannabis. They have helped thousands of people recover their wellbeing.

Caraway

Caraway is a very beneficial gut remedy for many conditions, and it is almost always used in combination with mint in research studies.[101] The actions of this powerful spice include antimicrobial, anti-inflammatory, antispasmodic, and antioxidant actions. Research shows that it helps reduce stomach pain and indigestion, reduce bloating, and more. It may even help normalize thyroid function and help reduce appetite in some people.[102]

Typically, between 25–50 mg of caraway oil combined with 20–40 mg of mint oil is used in research. [103]

Cardamom

I serendipitously came across a piece of cardamom's medical history at an antique store. Here, I found a medicine bottle labeled "Tinctura Cardamomi Composita." This is a blend of cardamom, cassia cinnamon, and caraway herbs that was described in the *King's American Dispensary* in the late 1800s

---

[101] Farhangi M, Dehghan P, et al. The effects of Nigella sativa on thyroid function, serum Vascular Endothelial Growth Factor (VEGF) - 1, Nesfatin-1 and anthropometric features in patients with Hashimoto's thyroiditis: a randomized controlled trial. *BMC Complement Altern Med.* 2016 Nov 16;16(1):471.

[102] Li J, Lv L, et al. A combination of peppermint oil and caraway oil for the treatment of functional dyspepsia: a systematic review and meta-analysis. *Evid Based Complement Alternat Med.* 2019 Nov 14;2019:7654947.

[103] Melchior C, Gourcerol G, et al. Efficacy of antibiotherapy for treating flatus incontinence associated with small intestinal bacterial overgrowth: A pilot randomized trial. *PLoS ONE.* 2017;12(8): e0180835.

and historically used for digestive ailments and lung disorders. This tincture was found on shelves in apothecaries up until Flexner came along.

Since the early recorded history of **Ayurvedic medicine**, cardamom has been used for its warming medicinal qualities. This effect brings balance back to the body when needed. Cardamom is useful for helping to treat acid reflux and reducing nausea, intestinal spasms, IBS, diarrhea, gas, constipation, gallbladder issues, and more. People also use cardamom for mental fatigue, loss of appetite, menstrual cramps, pancreatitis, colic, and more. It may even help protect the stomach from ulcers. I find cardamom very beneficial for minor belly aches and indigestion, and I just use a few fresh cardamom pods in hot water to make tea with it. Alternatively, you can buy cardamom capsules in doses of 500 mg, but very few brands sell them.

Catnip

If you think that catnip is just for cats, you are missing out. A close relative to mint, catnip grows vigorously in gardens and has relaxing effects for people too. It is easy to make catnip tea from fresh or dried leaves steeped in boiling water. It has long been used to help alleviate indigestion, for promoting a calm mood, and promotes sleep because it has similar properties to valerian root. A relaxed body and mind with healthy sleep promote healthy digestive function.

Chamomile

Well-known for its relaxing and sleep-promoting capabilities, chamomile also benefits your gut. It can help alleviate symptoms of diarrhea, gas, bloating, nausea, and upset stomach. I often drink chamomile along with other herbs in teas, but you can also get chamomile in capsule form as well. You can often find it with other relaxing herbs like valerian root, passionflower, holy basil, and skullcap.

Did You Know . . . Activated Charcoal is a Great Gut Remedy

Activated charcoal isn't an herb or spice but a remedy worth mentioning. This compound is made by exposing coconut shell fibers to high temperatures without oxygen to activate it. The heat processing makes charcoal porous and able to adsorb toxins in the gut but also absorb gas. This can be very helpful for reducing gut pain and also for helping to treat diarrhea. It also has very few side effects compared to standard anti-diarrheal medications.

Additionally, charcoal helps small intestinal bacterial overgrowth (SIBO) by helping alleviate abdominal pain. People with SIBO taking charcoal have less hydrogen gas production and better quality of life than those receiving antibiotics alone for this condition.[104]

Some people use activated charcoal as a digestion remedy after overindulging to reduce the toxic burden of unhealthier foods. Still, others feel like it helps them clear a food sensitivity exposure. For example, they recover from exposure to gluten much more quickly than without it.

Using activated charcoal reduces IBS symptoms, including constipation, by 60 percent. When given as a supplement called Nucarb, activated charcoal reduced the severity of constipation by 81 percent, straining by 72.69 percent, and incomplete evacuation by 72 percent.[105] Charcoal can cause constipation, but it usually happens when using high doses. You should know that charcoal is meant to be used occasionally, for a few days, and then take a break. You can learn more about activated charcoal in my blog post here: https://thehe althyrd.com/surprising-coconut-charcoal-benefits-for-gut-health-and-more/ High-quality activated charcoal is available in health food stores or on Fullscript.

---

[104] Ali R, Irfan M, et al. Efficacy of natural formulation containing activated charcoal, calcium sennosides, peppermint oil, fennel oil, rhubarb extract, and purified sulfur (Nucarb®) in relieving constipation. *Cureus.* 2021 Oct 1;13(10):e18419.

[105] Thompson A, Meah D, et al. Comparison of the antibacterial activity of essential oils and extracts of medicinal and culinary herbs to investigate potential new treatments for irritable bowel syndrome. *BMC Complement Altern Med.* 2013 Nov 28;13:338.

Coriander and Cilantro

One of my favorite spices is coriander seeds. Even for people who dislike cilantro, coriander seeds can be an appealing choice to cook with and use medicinally for gut health. Traditionally, coriander seeds are used for many ailments because they are rich in antioxidants and help balance the immune system. Research shows it helps reduce abdominal pain, bloating, and discomfort in people with IBS.[106] This is one that I like to maximize in my diet by cooking with it regularly, but you can certainly find supplements of coriander as well.

In contrast, cilantro leaves from the coriander plant are more well-known for their ability to bind and remove heavy metals from the body. Heavy metals are a much bigger problem for people than in the past due to air pollution, antibiotics and other medications, amalgam dental fillings, and contaminated fish. Heavy metals silently enter the body and cause lots of damage throughout the body, including the gut. There are case reports of people clearing their mercury toxicity by taking cilantro supplements and adopting other healthy lifestyle habits.[107]

Dill

You will be hard-pressed to find a research study about the benefits of dill for gut health, but like most herbs and spices, dill is rich in antioxidants that are great for the gut lining. Traditional uses of dill include the use for stimulating liver health, making digestive enzymes, and improving the flow

---

[106] Omura Y, Beckman S. Role of mercury (Hg) in resistant infections & effective treatment of Chlamydia trachomatis and Herpes family viral infections (and potential treatment for cancer) by removing localized Hg deposits with Chinese parsley and delivering effective antibiotics using various drug uptake enhancement methods. *Acupunct Electrother Res.* 1995 Aug–Dec;20(3-4):195–229.

[107] Thompson A, Meah D, et al. Comparison of the antibacterial activity of essential oils and extracts of medicinal and culinary herbs to investigate potential new treatments for irritable bowel syndrome. *BMC Complement Altern Med.* 2013 Nov 28;13:338.

of bile. Many people feel like they have less gas and bloating when eating dill, which is probably why.

Epazote

Epazote is an herb similar to Mexican oregano. This herb has reported benefits in reducing gas and bloating. Research shows that epazote can help eradicate intestinal parasites.[108] However, this herb is best used as a culinary herb unless under the supervision of a trained herbalist.

Fennel

When it comes to spices, fennel is a powerhouse, including reducing gas and bloating, decreasing IBS symptoms, reducing colic and abdominal spasms, helping both diarrhea and constipation, may reduce nausea, and may even reduce symptoms of acid reflux by promoting natural emptying of the stomach. It is also great for the liver and bile flow.

To use fennel, simply chew up ¼ to ½ teaspoon of fennel seeds after a meal. You can also take these seeds and put them in hot water for about 10 minutes to make tea. Many studies combine fennel with other spices like turmeric or anise.[109] [110] To learn more about fennel, read my blog post about it here: https://thehealthyrd.com/fennel-seeds-for-digestion/

---

[108] Madisch A, Holtmann G, et al. Treatment of irritable bowel syndrome with herbal preparations: results of a double-blind, randomized, placebo-controlled, multi-centre trial. *Aliment Pharmacol Ther.* 2004 Feb 1;19(3):271–9.

[109] Kliks M. Studies on the traditional herbal anthelmintic Chenopodium ambrosioides L.: ethnopharmacological evaluation and clinical field trials. *Soc Sci Med.* 1985;21(8):879–86.

[110] Ghodsi Z, Asltoghiri M. The effect of fennel on pain quality, symptoms, and menstrual duration in primary dysmenorrhea. *J Pediatr Adolesc Gynecol.* 2014 Oct;27(5):283–6.

Garlic

There is no question that garlic is a healthy ingredient for the whole body because its benefits are rooted in its immune-enhancing effects in the gut. It has powerful antimicrobial effects when eaten raw. It can also improve your microbiome's health because it contains plenty of prebiotic fiber. It is great for the liver and bile flow as well. Fermented garlic can even reduce the chances of getting colds and flu and lessens the symptoms when you do get sick. Used as part of the regimen for the natural treatment of small intestinal bacterial overgrowth, garlic is potent indeed.

However, some people are sensitive to garlic because it contains a carbo-hydrate called fructans. Personally, I love garlic for gut health, but it does result in some indigestion. If you get some indigestion from garlic, it is worth adding comprehensive digestive enzymes (see Chapter 5, page 54) to alleviate these symptoms.

Ginger

If you were to keep just one herb or spice around for digestive health, it should be ginger. But why limit yourself to just one when there are so many powerful ones? Ginger is the little spice that could because it contains over 100 compounds that heal the gut. It can alleviate just about every digestive condition imaginable. Containing natural digestive enzymes[111] and antioxidants[112] to cancer-preventing compounds,[113] ginger gets it done. From nausea to IBS and indigestion, most people find some relief quickly after eating ginger.

---

[111] Huang X, Chen L, et al. Purification, characterization, and milk coagulating properties of ginger proteases. *Journal of Dairy Science.* 2011:94(5): 2259–69.

[112] Bode A, Dong Z. The Amazing and Mighty Ginger. In: Benzie IFF, Wachtel-Galor S, editors. *Herbal Medicine: Biomolecular and Clinical Aspects.* 2nd edition. Boca Raton (FL): CRC Press/Taylor & Francis; 2011. Chapter 7.

[113] Kaur I, Deol P, et al. Anticancer Potential of Ginger: Mechanistic and Pharmacological Aspects. *Curr Pharm Des.* 2016;22(27):4160-72.

You can make ginger tea by steeping about ½ inch peeled root ginger in hot water for 5–10 minutes. Alternatively, add pickled ginger to your meal, grate fresh ginger into beverages, add ginger to recipes, and supplement with ginger capsules. Ginger candies are convenient too, but be careful because the added sugar can pile up if you use it all the time. If using ginger to alleviate digestive discomfort, I recommend having small amounts of fresh ginger every 15 minutes until your symptoms subside. I wrote an extensive blog about ginger's benefits, and you can access it here: https://thehealthyrd.com/12-amazing-benefits-of-ginger-for-digestion/

Iberogast

Iberogast is a blend of nine herbal extracts, and numerous clinical studies demonstrate its effectiveness in digestive conditions like dyspepsia, which many people think of as heartburn.[114] It does indeed help reduce symptoms of heartburn, improves muscle movements of the gut, reduces abdominal pain, and reduces symptoms of IBS. Because it has undeniable gut benefits, a major drug company called Bayer purchased Iberogast. Its herbs are bitter candytuft, chamomile, angelica root, caraway, milk thistle, lemon balm, peppermint, greater celandine, and licorice root.

Importantly, Iberogast has a much higher safety profile than conventional medications for these conditions. However, there have been a few rare side effects (less than twenty) of liver damage or other intolerances among the over 20 million users. For this reason, it is important that you follow the package directions and always get routine follow up with your doctor as you should anyway. You can buy Iberogast in many retail stores and online.

---

[114] Prasad S, Tyagi A. Ginger and its constituents: role in prevention and treatment of gastrointestinal cancer. *Gastroenterol Res Pract.* 2015;2015:142979.

Lavender

Lavender is usually thought of as a calming herb, but it has beneficial effects on the gut too. In fact, it may help reduce nausea and digestive pain as well as gas pain because it is rich in anti-inflammatory properties that calm the body. Many people even feel using lavender helps reduce anxiety more than conventional anxiety medications.

Did you know . . . Lemons ease nausea

While not technically an herb, lemon and its zest can be used medicinally like an herb, and it is so easy to use in a beverage or cooking. A major benefit of lemon is that the smell of it alone can reduce nausea. When we smell lemon, tiny lemon molecules are dissolved in the nasal cavity. This then stimulates neurons that give messages to the brain to dampen nausea.

Limonene from lemons taken orally may be protective against stomach ulcers, and it also increases gastric mucus, a protective layer of the stomach. Surprisingly, lemon may even be a natural alternative for heartburn. Patients receiving 1 g of limonene daily from lemons found relief from heartburn. In fact, 89 percent had a complete resolution of heartburn symptoms after fourteen days of using limonene.[115] [116] While this was a small sponsored study, I recommend that you read about limonene supplement reviews to learn how people find it beneficial for their heartburn. One small study even

---

[115] Ottillinger B, Storr M, et al. STW 5 (Iberogast®)—a safe and effective standard in the treatment of functional gastrointestinal disorders. *Wien Med Wochenschr.* 2013 Feb;163(3-4):65–72.

[116] von Arnim U, Peitz U, et al. STW 5, a phytopharmacon for patients with functional dyspepsia: results of a multicenter, placebo-controlled double-blind study. *Am J Gastroenterol.* 2007 Jun;102(6):1268–75.

showed that lemon essential oil may reduce gallstones. [117] [118]

Lemon Balm

Like mint, lemon balm is a vigorously growing plant that smells and tastes like lemon. As is commonly found in edible herbs, lemon balm is rich in antioxidants that help calm the nervous system and support digestive health. While research is scant about lemon balm's effectiveness for gut health, some show it helps reduce symptoms of dyspepsia, indigestion, and heartburn.[119] The German Commission E recommends lemon balm as a treatment for many digestive ailments too. It is also generally recognized as safe. [120] [121]

Lemon balm makes a great tea infusion that is relaxing. Of note, it is one of the herbs in the beneficial Iberogast supplement listed above.

Licorice

Licorice is a very powerful herb for the gut, and because of this, it also needs special consideration when using it. Several clinical studies show that it works as well or better than proton pump inhibitors for acid reflux,

---

[117] Willette R, Barrow L, et al. Purified d-limonene: An effective agent for the relief of occasional symptoms of heartburn. Proprietary study. WRC Laboratories, Inc. Galveston, TX.

[118] Igimi H, Hisatsugu T, et al The use of d-limonene preparation as a dissolving agent of gallstones. Am J Dig Dis. 1976 Nov;21(11):926-39.

[119] Ulbricht C, Brendler T, et al. Natural Standard Research Collaboration. Lemon balm (Melissa officinalis L.): an evidence-based systematic review by the Natural Standard Research Collaboration. J Herb Pharmacother. 2005;5(4):71-114.

[120] Lemon Balm - American Botanical Council, https://www.herbalgram.org/resources/expanded-commission-e/lemon-balm/.

[121] Raveendra K, Jayachandra, et al. An Extract of Glycyrrhiza glabra (GutGard) Alleviates Symptoms of Functional Dyspepsia: A Randomized, Double-Blind, Placebo-Controlled Study. Evid Based Complement Alternat Med. 2012;2012:216970.

indigestion, and for reducing stomach ulcers. [122] [123]Adding licorice to standard treatment for **H. pylori** infections of the stomach also improves the response to antibiotic therapy[124] and also works great to help alleviate nausea.

However, licorice has a compound called glycyrrhizin that can increase **cortisol** levels, reduce blood potassium levels and cause an increase in blood pressure. This is especially true if you use licorice daily. To be safe, it is best to use de-glycyrrhizinate (DGL) licorice if you use it regularly. A good DGL supplement can be found in health food stores or Fullscript.

Marshmallow Root

Marshmallow root is a favorite herb of mine because it is very gentle, and you can think of it as a warm blanket for the gut lining. It is rich in mucin, which protects the gut lining, with countless reports of its healing effects. Ancient Egyptians used marshmallow root to ease coughs and heal wounds too.

Marshmallow extract stimulates the growth of gut cells and makes them less leaky, according to some research.[125] [126] So, not only is marshmallow root good for the intestines, but it is also helpful if you struggle with acid reflux, gastric ulcers, and GERD because it's so protective.

---

[122] Di Pierro F, Gatti M, et al. Outcomes in patients with nonerosive reflux disease treated with a proton pump inhibitor and alginic acid ± glycyrrhetinic acid and anthocyanosides. Clin Exp Gastroenterol. 2013;6:27-33.

[123] Hajiaghamohammadi A, Zargar A, et al. To evaluate of the effect of adding licorice to the standard treatment regimen of Helicobacter pylori. Braz J Infect Dis. 2016 Nov-Dec;20(6):534-538.

[124] Jalilzadeh-Amin G, Najarnezhad V, et al. Antiulcer properties of Glycyrrhiza glabra L. extract on experimental models of gastric ulcer in mice. Iran J Pharm Res. 2015 Fall;14(4):1163-70.

[125] Zaghlool S, Shehata B, et al. Protective effects of ginger and marshmallow extracts on indomethacin-induced peptic ulcer in rats. *J Nat Sci Biol Med.* 2015 Jul-Dec;6(2):421–8.

[126] Deters A, Zippel J, et al. Aqueous extracts and polysaccharides from Marshmallow roots (Althea officinalis L.): cellular internalisation and stimulation of cell physiology of human epithelial cells in vitro. *J Ethnopharmacol.* 2010 Jan 8;127(1):62–9.

You can buy marshmallow root at health food stores and make tea with it or use a high-quality marshmallow root supplement in health food stores or on Fullscript.

Milk Thistle

Many people feel better during bouts of IBS when taking milk thistle (Silybum marianum), even though there is no direct research to prove this link. This is likely because milk thistle helps reduce gas and bloating and balances the microbiome. Much research has demonstrated that milk thistle is a safe and effective treatment for liver issues,[127] and because it does this, it also tends to help digestive function. As you may recall, the liver is responsible for making bile which helps your body digest fats and vitamins.

Using milk thistle can help make the bowels more regular. And like many herbs, milk thistle also helps to improve antioxidant levels and reduce inflammation in the intestines, according to early research.[128] [129] [130]

You can make milk thistle tea from herbal stores or take milk thistle supplements from Fullscript. For more information about milk thistle, read my blog post at https://thehealthyrd.com/milk-thistle-for-ibs-liver-health-and-more/.

---

[127] Abenavoli L, Capasso R, et al. Milk thistle in liver diseases: past, present, future. *Phytother Res.* 2010 Oct;24(10):1423-32.

[128] Al-hazmi A, Alomery A, et al. Silymarin as a therapeutic extract for intestinal and splenic injuries induced by microcystin-LR in mice. *Journal of King Saud University – Science.* 2019 31(4): 1414–17.

[129] Zhong S, Fan Y, et al. The therapeutic effect of silymarin in the treatment of nonalcoholic fatty disease: A meta-analysis (PRISMA) of randomized control trials. *Medicine (Baltimore).* 2017 Dec;96(49):e9061.

[130] Shen L, Liu L, et al. Regulation of gut microbiota in Alzheimer's disease mice by silibinin and silymarin and their pharmacological implications. *Appl Microbiol Biotechnol.* 2019 Sep;103(17):7141–9.

Peppermint

One of the first things I was taught in college nutrition classes is that peppermint can increase the risk of reflux, not its amazingly healing properties, sadly. Even sadder is that mint can benefit acid reflux and reduce dyspepsia symptoms according to some research. It is an important ingredient in the supplement for dyspepsia called Iberogast. Research even shows that it can be helpful for babies who struggle with colic.[131]

Here is a short list of some of the peppermint's gut-healing effects:

- Anti-inflammatory
- Reduces the growth of candida
- Protects against E. coli
- Reduces nausea
- Reduces IBS symptoms
- Relaxes gut smooth muscles by its direct enteric nervous symptom effects
- Reduces gas and bloating
- Supports a healthy gallbladder
- Reduces dyspepsia

Peppermint is easy to find and use, provided you are not sensitive to it. However, pay attention to its quality and dosing instructions for each condition because it is possible to overdo it.

Mullein

Although mullein (*Verbascum thapsus*) is most well-known for its lung health benefits, it has multiple benefits, including for gut health. While research related to gut health and mullein continues to be scant, it has anti-

---

[131] Alves J, de Brito Rde C, et al. Effectiveness of mentha piperita in the treatment of infantile colic: a crossover study. *Evid Based Complement Alternat Med.* 2012;2012:981352.

inflammatory, anti-parasitic effects, and muscle-relaxing effects. It also helps fight harmful gut bugs, like E. coli and Klebsiella pneumoniae.

Traditional uses also included its uses for ability to help treat gallstones, constipation, and gut inflammation. Mullein tea is safe to drink 3–4 times daily. And if you do have lung issues, I highly suggest that you research its benefits, as people report recovering from daunting lung issues by using this herb.

Oregano

Oregano is a potent culinary herb with powerful effects that help regulate the gut microbiome. Used in small amounts, it can easily be incorporated into many culinary dishes and is very safe. Powerful enough to even help treat small intestinal bacterial overgrowth and candida overgrowth, oregano is a tool many people can use to help their digestive function.

When used in teas and in foods, oregano is a great herb that boosts the immune system, protects from free radicals, and more. It is also safe for very short-term digestive ailments. For example, I find it is great for nausea and indigestion. Gaia makes a nice variety of oregano oil, and you can find it at any reputable store or on Fullscript. However, because oregano is so potent in supplement form, it is best to be used under the supervision of a qualified naturopath or functional medicine doctor for more challenging chronic conditions like small intestinal bacterial overgrowth and candida overgrowth.

Red Raspberry Leaf

Red raspberry leaf is an unsung hero for hormonal and female health, but it is also great for calming the gut. The deer in my garden devour it, so they must know something most people don't know! It is also excellent that you are looking for a natural way to reduce diarrhea symptoms. Many users describe red raspberry leaf as a great support for regular bowel movements.

One word for red raspberry leaf that sums it up: balancing. Containing lots of antioxidants, raspberry leaves dampen inflammation in the gut and are gentle enough to use daily. Drinking raspberry leaf tea is a popular way to get it into your diet.

However, you should avoid using red raspberry leaf if you are pregnant, although it can be great to use in the days leading up to your estimated due date to help encourage labor. It is also wonderful for reducing menstrual cramps. Alternatively, you can find red raspberry leaf supplements at any reputable store or Fullscript.

Slippery Elm

Slippery elm has an interesting history. People have used it as a food source when food is scarce during starvation. Baseball players even used to chew slippery elm because it enhanced saliva production for spitballs back in the day. Because it increases saliva production, you probably can also guess it helps digestion. Its ability to increase mucus secretion in the esophagus and stomach protects the gut. It also helps to regulate bowel movements by bringing water into the gut and adding bulk to the stool as well. Owing to its anti-inflammatory effects, it also is likely good for people with inflammatory bowel diseases.

This medicinal plant is generally considered safe, but if you are on prescription medications, it is best to take them two hours before using slippery elm. Slippery elm is often combined with marshmallow root because of their similar actions.

Senna

Senna is a safe and effective herb for gut issues, especially constipation. However, there is a lot of misinformation about it on the internet and otherwise. A review of eight clinical studies in children concluded that senna is safe for use and only causes an occasional rash for sensitive people.[132]

Unlike conventional over-the-counter laxatives, senna is helpful for the gut because it also has antioxidant effects. Contrary to popular belief, it is not addicting or habit-forming. However, you should avoid large doses, as there are rare case reports of people consuming a large amount that resulted in the temporary elevation of liver enzymes. Generally, doses of less than 15 mg per day of senna are safe.

Stone Breaker Herb

Stone breaker (*chanca piedra*) herb may help with exactly what it is nicknamed to do—reduce the risk of gallstones and kidney stones. Research shows that it helps to reduce the size of kidney stones,[133] and it doesn't have toxic effects. Traditional medicine uses of stone breaker are also for gallstones. It makes sense that it may help for this condition because it reduces inflammation and naturally reduces pain and the growth of harmful bacteria.

It is usually taken in tincture form, 1–2 drops per day initially and increasing up to 30–40 drops per day before meals being a common serving size per day. It is available on Fullscript or from health food stores.

Thyme

Similar to the potent oregano herb, thyme (*Thymus vulgaris*) is used frequently to curb the growth of harmful bacteria and excess candida yeast. Using thyme is a great culinary herb that supports immune and gut functions because of its anti-inflammatory effects.

Often combined with fenugreek, this combination is most often used for its respiratory and allergy benefits. But, as you can imagine, these conditions

---

[132] Vilanova-Sanchez A, Gasior A, et al. Are Senna based laxatives safe when used as long term treatment for constipation in children? *J Pediatr Surg.* 2018 Apr;53(4):722–7.

[133] Lee N, Khoo W, et al. The pharmacological potential of Phyllanthus niruri. *J Pharm Pharmacol.* 2016;68(8):953–69.

are often rooted in gut imbalances, and this is part of why they are so helpful in these conditions.

You can make thyme tea, a super inexpensive drink, using it this way. Alternatively, you can find thyme supplements on Fullcript or in health food stores.

Tulsi

Tulsi, also known as holy basil, is an herb that is an adaptogen that helps calm the body while also promoting healthy energy levels. It's a favorite tea in many countries and has become a staple in my daily routine. It tastes great, especially with herbs like rose, chai spices, or ginger.

Tulsi reduces stress and anxiety, according to clinical studies.[134] Fascinatingly, it also may help improve memory and have neuroprotective effects. My favorite way to use tulsi is to drink tulsi tea. You can also get tulsi in capsule form here, and a typical dose is 900 mg per day.

Turmeric

Turmeric is probably the most popular medicinal plant supplement today because it has proven benefits for reducing joint aches and pains as it dampens inflammation. Still, it also is known to improve the microbiome

[134] Saxena R, Singh R, et al. Efficacy of an extract of ocimum tenuiflorum (OciBest) in the Management of general stress: A double-blind, placebo-controlled study. *Evid Based Complement Alternat Med.* 2012;2012:894509.

balance, so it definitely can be very good for gut health.[135] [136] [137]

As with anything with potent health benefits, some risks can be associated. I know several people who developed some gut pain when using turmeric. I'll say it again: it's important to remember that what is good for one person is not always good for the next. Still, most people find turmeric very beneficial for overall health. Because it is so popular, you can find turmeric supplements everywhere. However, quality can vary significantly.

As a rule, eat turmeric during a meal that has a good amount of fat in it to optimize its tolerance and absorption. Even better yet, cook turmeric with meals that have butter, extra virgin olive oil, or butter to enhance its taste and effectiveness. You can supplement turmeric as well as many people, but again, it will work better with a healthy meal.

Triphala

Triphala is a blend of plants that are stress-busting but also very good for the gut. Containing *Emblica officinalis, Terminalia bellerica*, and *Terminalia chebula,* which are native to India. High in antioxidants, Triphala helps support intestinal protein content while damping inflammation in the intestinal wall. Using Triphala improves constipation and eases abdominal pain, dyspepsia, and gas while promoting increased regularity of bowel movements, according to research.[138] You can find triphala in health food

[135] Scazzocchio B, Minghetti L, et al. Interaction between gut microbiota and curcumin: A new key of understanding for the health effects of curcumin. *Nutrients.* 2020 Aug 19;12(9):2499.

[136] Munshi R, Bhalerao S, et al. An open-label, prospective clinical study to evaluate the efficacy and safety of TLPL/AY/01/2008 in the management of functional constipation. *J Ayurveda Integr Med.* 2011 Jul;2(3):144–52.

[137] Mukherjee P, Rai S, et al. (2006). Clinical study of "triphala" – A well known phytomedicine from India. *Iranian Journal of Pharmacology and Therapeutics* (ISSN: 1735-2657) Vol 5 Num 1. 5.

[138] Nariya M, Shukla V, et al. Comparison of enteroprotective efficacy of triphala formulations (Indian Herbal Drug) on methotrexate-induced small intestinal damage in rats. *Phytother Res.* 2009 Aug;23(8):1092–8.

stores or on Fullscript.

8

Chapter 8

The Magical Properties of Probiotics and Prebiotics

Probiotics are any live or dormant microorganisms intentionally introduced to improve wellbeing. They are primarily used for gut health, but that hasn't stopped the research from discovering their many bodily roles. This is because there is cross-talk between the gut microbiome and every tissue in your system.[139]

In contrast, prebiotics is a much newer area of treatment protocols and help feed probiotics to help them take up residence in the gut. They are primarily in the form of fermentable fibers, as reviewed in Chapter 6. Vitamins and minerals also fuel probiotics, so they can have prebiotic-like effects too.

Probiotics and prebiotics have become so popular. In fact, around a third of the United States population use them regularly, and you are probably familiar with them. So, while this chapter may be a review for you, there are also some ways to use probiotics that may surprise you here. In the following chapters, I will explore how various probiotics and prebiotics fit

---

[139] Martínez J, Vargas A, Pérez-Sánchez T, et al. Human microbiota network: Unveiling potential crosstalk between the different microbiota ecosystems and their role in health and disease. *Nutrients*. 2021 Aug 24;13(9):2905.

into treatment regimens of all kinds for the gut and how to use them.

Probiotics Overview

The science of probiotics has exploded in recent years, and there isn't a health condition that truly isn't affected by them to some degree. The understanding that everything in the body is connected via the gut is not only truly remarkable, but it also changes lives daily. That's not to say that probiotics are a one-size-fits-all approach; nothing could be further from the truth. Your gut microbiome, which is host to your own probiotic environment, will have a unique response to the hundreds of strains of probiotics.

Your microbiome is uniquely you, and no two microbiomes are alike. Still, there are enough commonalities between gut microbiomes that certain strains help with certain health conditions no matter who you are.

Did You Know . . . Research into Probiotics Is a Hot Topic

If you search the Library of Medicine for probiotic strains for any health condition, you will find a rich body of research beginning to emerge.[140] Some conditions have a lot of evidence behind them, as is in the case of probiotics for anxiety and depression. Certain probiotics like *Lactobacillus rhamnosus* are even effective in helping to prevent recurrent urinary tract infections. And while you may not think of probiotics if you suffer from acid reflux, you should. The research shows that out of thirteen clinical studies, 79 percent show that probiotics are an effective treatment strategy for acid reflux.[141]

Every gut condition that exists today has been studied in relation to how probiotics may or may not work. In the following chapters, you will learn

---

[140] Martínez J, Vargas A, Pérez-Sánchez T, et al. Human microbiota network: unveiling potential crosstalk between the different microbiota ecosystems and their role in health and disease. *Nutrients.* 2021 Aug 24;13(9):2905.

[141] Probiotics - Search Results - Pubmed. National Center for Biotechnology Information, U.S. National Library of Medicine, https://pubmed.ncbi.nlm.nih.gov/?term=probiotics.

how various conditions may benefit from certain probiotic strains. But, you should always keep in mind that you are unique, and so your response to them also may be unique. Some other areas, aside from gut benefits, where probiotics are proving helpful include:

- Treating acne
- Improving sleep quality
- Bad breath
- Reducing eczema and psoriasis
- Liver health
- Reducing high blood pressure and high cholesterol
- Reducing blood sugar levels in people with diabetes

Luckily, there is very little to be harmed and a lot to be gained by considering probiotics as a daily part of your diet or in supplement form. That said, there is an exception; if you are severely immune compromised, such as if you are hospitalized with an immunological condition, have pancreatitis, or receiving cancer treatment, you should use caution with probiotic supplements. And, because we are all so different, you may find those very popular probiotics may cause some mild side effects, such as digestive distress, while other less common strains may be beneficial and have no side effects. It takes some trial and error, so I encourage you to keep a journal of the strains and brands that you try so that you can make an educated decision based on your own individual response. Finding the right probiotics is well worth your time if you don't foresee eating fermented foods daily, as most people don't do this.

Most Common Probiotic Strains

Here are the most common genus of probiotic strains and how they function in the body.

Bacillus

Bacillus bacteria are naturally found in the soil and are also called soil-based or spore-based probiotics. This means they are inactive when you take them but become active in your gut. For this reason, they are much less likely than others to have negative side effects in the small intestine. Although much less common than other probiotic types, Bacillus strains have become my favorite to recommend and use for myself and my family.

The Bacillus genus not only serves as probiotics, but they also help the body to break down food. For example, resistant starches from your food are broken down by Bacillus, which makes them easier to digest. Once these starches are broken down, they become prebiotics too. So really, Bacillus serves both as probiotics and prebiotics in a sense. And by becoming prebiotics, the starches they transform help to feed the healthy bacteria that live in your gut.

The friendly bacteria made by soil probiotics include Akkermansia. This fascinating type of resident probiotic is known to help restore the gut lining, help overall digestive health, and is even helpful for weight loss. Friendly bacteria like Akkermansia help to prevent leaky gut and boost metabolism.

Strains of Bacillus probiotics include Bacillus coagulans, Bacillus clausii, Bacillus subtilis, Bacillus licheniformis, and Bacillus indicus. One huge perk of taking spore-based probiotics is that a low dose, often around 2–5 billion spore-based probiotics, is enough to have benefits. This is another reason why they are very well-tolerated. However, the breadth of understanding of probiotics remains with Lactobacillus and Bifidobacterium types of probiotics. This doesn't mean that spore-based are any less effective- it just means they have had less time and attention devoted to them in research.

Bifidobacterium

Bifidobacterium is a type of bacteria becoming very common in various probiotic blends. This genus of probiotics is often helpful if struggling with taking *Lactobacillus* strains because Bifidobacterium does not cause a release of histamine in the body like some Lactobacillus strains.

Bifidobacterium is helpful for functional dyspepsia, GERD, overall digestive distress and pain, reduces constipation and diarrhea symptoms, and increases stomach emptying speed. Some strains of Bifidobacterium, such as Bifidobacterium longum, may be useful in helping to treat daunting conditions like inflammatory bowel diseases. Not surprisingly, they also help the body by preventing opportunistic infections like H. pylori and rotavirus and reducing the severity of colds and upper respiratory infections. Bifidobacterium is also likely useful in helping prevent and treat seasonal allergies.

Additionally, Bifidobacterium produces fuel for your gut by making compounds called short-chain fatty acids like butyrate. However, if you have SIBO, you are more likely to have negative symptoms from Bifidobacterium because some strains, such as Bifidobacterium lactis, may increase the production of gasses like methane in the small intestine.

Unlike Bacillus strains, Bifidobacterium probiotics are usually more effective at higher doses and in multi-strain combinations. So, for example, you are more likely to find benefit if you find a high-dose probiotic with greater than 20 billion strains with multiple types of Bifidobacterium and/or Lactobacillus.

Lactobacillus

By far, the most common types of probiotic on the market today are Lactobacillus. These live organisms have been around the longest in terms of probiotic supplements, and for this reason, they have the most research about them. Used far and wide for almost every health condition, Lactobacillus strains are diverse and helpful for so many aspects of health. These natural bacteria are found in fermented foods like sauerkraut and pickled vegetables.

Due to Lactobacillus' wide reach for their health effects, you can imagine they help with mood, prevent infections, reduce a multitude of gut issues, and may help improve liver function, gallbladder health, skin health, and much more.

Even though they are the most common, Lactobacillus is sometimes a culprit for some GI side effects, which are usually temporary. They also can increase histamine production, so Lactobacillus may not be the first choice if you have an intolerance.

When you take a probiotic with Lactobacillus strains, the variety of strains and the amount matter. For example, you will usually want at least 20 billion CFUs and as many strains as possible to get the best chance of a benefit. These days, they are often combined with Bifidobacterium strains too, which is a good thing.

If you have SIBO, it is best to choose your strain carefully, and research shows that Lactobacillus rhamnosus, Lactobacillus acidophilus, and Lacto-bacillus reuteri is your best bets.[142]

Saccharomyces

Saccharomyces boulardii is a live yeast type of probiotic, making it unique. It doesn't reside in the gut, typically used short-term for specific health conditions. The nice thing to remember about Saccharomyces is that it has been used for decades safely for many purposes.

This type of probiotic only has one strain, so it is easier to remember than most—Saccharomyces boulardii. It does many things to help with health, including supporting the immune system and keeping the gut in balance by strengthening the gut lining. Saccharomyces boulardii also helps the body absorb nutrients. This is important for anyone with SIBO or any inflammatory bowel condition, as they cannot absorb nutrients.

---

[142] Cheng J, Ouwehand A. Gastroesophageal reflux disease and probiotics: a systematic review. nutrients. 2020 Jan 2;12(1):132.

For specific conditions that Saccharomyces benefits, you should know that it reduces SIBO symptoms and other conditions, including diarrhea, abdominal pain, bloating, inflammatory bowel diseases, and IBS, reducing breath hydrogen levels. It is very effective in reducing antibiotic-associated diarrhea as well. Even more, Saccharomyces has also helped eradicate SIBO in some research studies.[143] [144] For these reasons, it is often considered one of the best probiotic strains. This is because Saccharomyces doesn't overgrow in the small bowel and doesn't take up residence. Make sure you choose a reputable brand with a live and active culture. You will most often find this strain as a stand-alone probiotic because of its stability. The other nice thing about this strain is that you don't need super-high doses. Research shows that doses between 10–20 billion CFUs daily are effective for adults. You can find Saccharomyces boulardii on Fullscript.

Advisory: Contraindications

It cannot be stressed enough if you are severely immunocompromised, such as with people undergoing chemotherapy, radiotherapy, or immunosuppressive drugs, you should not take Saccharomyces. Otherwise, *Saccharomyces* is a very safe type of probiotic to use with no side effects typically reported.

Prebiotics and Fiber, a Mixed Bag

Before diving into prebiotics and fiber, you should know that there are many good and possible bad effects of these compounds in the gut. Regarding prebiotics, the lines continue to be blurred because, as science expands its knowledge of this topic, the more we find that many types of fiber serve

---

[143] Kwak D, Jun D, et al. Short-term probiotic therapy alleviates small intestinal bacterial overgrowth, but does not improve intestinal permeability in chronic liver disease. *Eur J Gastroenterol Hepatol.* 2014 Dec;26(12):1353–9.

[144] Ojetti V, Petruzziello C, et al. Effect of *Lactobacillus reuteri* (DSM 17938) on methane production in patients affected by functional constipation: a retrospective study. *Eur Rev Med Pharmacol Sci.* 2017 Apr;21(7):1702–8. PMID: 28429333.

as prebiotics. The topic is so new, in fact, that the established function of prebiotics was established in 2016.[145] To sum up, a prebiotic is anything that helps selectively promote the growth and health of your microbiome. This typically means that prebiotics is certain kinds of fibers and nutrients. However, for some unknown reason, the official definition of prebiotics excludes dietary influences that affect the microbiome that isn't fiber-based, such as vitamins and minerals. Even though vitamins and minerals, even protein, can have prebiotic-like effects. So, for clarity, prebiotics is fermentable fibers that support gut microbiome health. However, not all fibers are fermentable, and not all fermentation in the gut is beneficial.

In my experience, prebiotics can be very beneficial but tricky to work with, especially if you struggle with gas and bloating. Just yesterday, I combined prebiotic food sources for lunch and had really bad gut pain. It wasn't a usual combination of foods, but I will never do that again—a whole avocado and a drink with inulin fiber. I usually respond well to some kinds of prebiotics, but like anything, the dose and your own individuality can make a poison. I basically ate too much of a good thing, and it turned into a pretty painful experience. So you see, you really need to be careful in this area.

Did You Know . . . Prebiotics Can Be Challenging

The challenge of getting prebiotic fibers in your diet is that they can also come from gut-triggering foods in other ways. For example, legumes and whole wheat are rich in prebiotic fibers but are the biggest culprits for gut pain. In fact, some research even shows that legumes and wheat can be causal in conditions like IBS and inflammatory bowel diseases.[146] And if there are foods that almost always cause gut pain for many of us, it's legumes and

---

[145] García-Collinot G, Madrigal-Santillán E, et al. Effectiveness of *Saccharomyces boulardii* and metronidazole for small intestinal bacterial overgrowth in systemic sclerosis. *Dig Dis Sci.* 2020 Apr;65(4):1134–43.

[146] Gibson G, Hutkins R, et al. Expert consensus document: the International Scientific Association for Probiotics and Prebiotics (ISAPP) consensus statement on the definition and scope of prebiotics. *Nat Rev Gastroenterol Hepatol.* 2017; 14, 491–502.

wheat. It doesn't matter how they are cooked, soaked, sprouted, or organic. I've tried all the ways. If I eat them one day, I'm usually fine, but if I have them a second or third day, I'm in misery. Research shows I'm not alone, and many people struggle with these two so-called healthy foods.[147] [148]

So with prebiotics, you are often comparing apples to oranges, and what you tolerate may be entirely different than the next person. The point I'm trying to make is that not all prebiotic fibers are good for everyone, and you should tread lightly on the amount of prebiotics, especially if you aren't used to them.

That said, there are some fairly gentle prebiotic fibers that most people tolerate and that are beneficial to people who typically have constipation and diarrhea, such as acacia fiber. My first fiber choices for IBS-D are acacia fiber, followed by guar gum, beta-glucan, and psyllium. Some people also do great with chicory fiber or inulin, but this one needs a slow introduction for many because it can ramp up gas and bloat. Generally, avoid flaxseed fiber unless you know for sure that you don't bloat up like a balloon from it or ferment it first before eating it.

Garlic, onions, leeks, asparagus, bananas, Jerusalem artichoke, avocados, oats, sweet potatoes, jicama, seaweed, and many other foods are naturally rich in prebiotics. Of these, bananas, sweet potatoes, jicama, and seaweed are often less likely to cause stomach upset.

After all these cautions, many people really can benefit from prebiotics, especially in promoting regularity. If you take a supplement for diarrhea or constipation symptoms, I recommend starting with the lowest dose possible, such as 2 g acacia fiber daily. This is 1 teaspoon of acacia fiber. Or you can use half the recommended dose listed on the supplement label.

---

[147] Pimental M, Rezaie Ali. *The Microbiome Connection* (1st ed.). 2022. Agate.
    Hayes P, Fraher M, et al. Irritable bowel syndrome: The role of food in pathogenesis and management. *Gastroenterol Hepatol* (N Y). 2014 Mar;10(3):164–74.

[148] Pimental M, Rezaie Ali. *The Microbiome Connection* (1st ed.). 2022. Agate.
    Hayes P, Fraher M, et al. Irritable bowel syndrome: The role of food in pathogenesis and management. *Gastroenterol Hepatol* (N Y). 2014 Mar;10(3):164–74.

Synbiotics Overview

The terminology synbiotics is relatively new, so I wanted to explain what it means if you haven't come across it. Synbiosis essentially means that the sum is equal to more than its parts. Synbiotics in the diet and supplements are foods and nutrients combined with synergistic effects on the gut. Examples of this might be yogurt and bananas or raw sauerkraut and avocado.

You will often see synbiotics listed on probiotics supplements because they combine probiotics and prebiotics. They are designed this way to promote the survivability of probiotic bacteria in the gut. But make sure to read the cautions about prebiotics before you choose a supplement that is considered a synbiotic.

Although there is a lot of marketing of these products, most symbiotic supplements contain such a marginal amount of prebiotics that it is unknown if they truly have symbiotic effects.

Postbiotics Overview

Postbiotics are the leftover byproducts of probiotics and prebiotics in the gut that can have powerfully beneficial effects on the body. Postbiotics include amino acids, dead bacterial pieces, short-chain fatty acids (butyrate), antimicrobial peptides, digestive enzymes, and vitamins. Because these compounds are so varied, they can also affect the body. An interesting aspect of postbiotics is that they benefit the immune system even after probiotics have died in the body. For this reason, probiotics that are taken that have passed on, so to speak, even benefit your body.

Research is beginning to show that some postbiotics like butyrate can have beneficial effects on the gut by reducing abdominal pain and symptoms in people who have IBS and Crohn's disease. Butyrate may even reduce the risk of GI infections.[149] [150]

I'm a huge fan of taking amino acids as postbiotic supplements. Amino acids that are considered postbiotics include tryptophan and tyrosine. These two compounds are critical for making mood-enhancing compounds in the gut, including serotonin and dopamine. In fact, when I started taking a combination of tryptophan and tyrosine, as recommended by Dr. Amen,[151] my mood has been improved greatly and never dipped.

Some argue that our body can make enough serotonin and dopamine from tryptophan and tyrosine in the diet. Still, research indicates that because of the chemical use of glyphosate that is so widespread, our ability to break down protein into these amino acids and then have them become serotonin and dopamine is impaired.[152] [153] While this is a big topic and a bit beyond the scope of this book, I highly recommend checking out Dr. Amen's website BrainMD at https://brainmd.com/. He has changed so many people's lives for the better, including mine. I truly wouldn't be where I am today without his advice. You can find butyrate supplements on Fullscript or in health food stores.

[149] Tuck C, Biesiekierski J, et al. Food intolerances. *Nutrients.* 2019 Jul 22;11(7):1684.
Limketkai B, Sepulveda R, et al. Prevalence and factors associated with gluten sensitivity in inflammatory bowel disease. *Scand J Gastroenterol.* 2018 Feb;53(2):147–51.

[150] García-Collinot G, Madrigal-Santillán et al. Effectiveness of *Saccharomyces boulardii* and metronidazole for small intestinal bacterial overgrowth in systemic sclerosis. *Dig Dis Sci.* 2020 Apr;65(4):1134–43.

[151] Banasiewicz T, Krokowicz Ł, e al. Microencapsulated sodium butyrate reduces the frequency of abdominal pain in patients with irritable bowel syndrome. Colorectal Dis. 2013 Feb;15(2):204–9.

[152] Amen Clinics. Transforming the way mental health is treated. mental healthcare clinic focusing on your brain health. https://www.amenclinics.com/.

[153] Samsel A, Seneff S. Glyphosate, pathways to modern diseases III: Manganese, neurological diseases, and associated pathologies. *Surg Neurol Int.* 2015 Mar 24;6:45.

Case Study: Gut Healing with Surprising Mood Benefits

Brian suffered from IBS, anxiety, and moodiness for years, and conventional medications resulted in more side effects than benefits. On advice from his doctor, he also began limiting high FODMAPS foods like beans, wheat, some fruits, and vegetables, too. The new diet helped his symptoms but didn't come close to eliminating them.

Frustrated with the lack of benefits, and on my advice, he started eating more healing foods—such as beef liver, salmon, cooked greens, root vegetables, fermented vegetables, and taking a broad-spectrum natural multivitamin with minerals along with extra vitamin D3 and vitamin K2. He continued to limit trigger foods, including legumes and wheat, as much as possible. He also started taking butyrate, which helped his bowels become more regular and significantly reduced his gut pain.

With butyrate's success, Brian was willing to try other postbiotics—tyrosine and tryptophan. Almost immediately, his mood was lighter, he was less negative, and he could even enjoy his favorite hobbies again, including playing music. Adding tyrosine and tryptophan also reduced his anxiety so much that he felt he didn't have it anymore. He continues to feel the benefits of the diet and supplement changes years later and won't go on vacation or a day without them. The amazing part is that he didn't get any side effects from taking the supplements and changing his diet, but he did get plenty of benefits.

9

Chapter 9

Heartburn: Finding Relief

This may be hard to believe, but heartburn and acid reflux are often easier digestive issues to fix with diet and supplements. By learning about the root cause of your condition, you can often fix it with some straightforward changes.

In this chapter, we will review what heartburn is, what can cause it, why conventional treatment often doesn't fix the problem, why stomach acid is critical for health, how to tell if you have low stomach acid, diet tips for reducing heartburn symptoms, and supplements that can help prevent and alleviate heartburn altogether.

What Is Heartburn and What Causes It

Acid reflux, also called heartburn, is simply a feeling of pain from undigested food and stomach fluids in the esophagus. It is most often due to digestive and food imbalances. Sometimes you might also feel abdominal pain with heartburn. What may seem like a condition caused by acid, heartburn usually starts with feelings of indigestion, which means that food isn't digesting well. Indigestion can result in belching, tasting your food hours after eating them, and general gut "yuck" feelings. Eventually, this indigestion leads to the classical burning sensation of heartburn if left unchecked.

The root cause of heartburn is often indigestion of foods due to a lack of healthy gut probiotics, lack of stomach acid (yes, you heard that right), lack of digestive enzymes, and a lack of nutrients that help the gut wall function properly.

All these feelings of indigestion and acid reflux are a red flag that you didn't eat right, or your gut isn't equipped with the right gear to deal with the food you've eaten. Think about it: eating donuts followed by a big soda will not end well for your stomach. Not surprisingly, there are almost no essential vitamins, minerals, enzymes, fiber, or probiotics that promote digestion in these foods. Even worse, these junk foods are full of inflammatory compounds that slow digestive function and worsen the condition of your stomach. Eating these indulgent types of foods also throws off the acid balance of the stomach and intestines and even throws off the ability to digest these foods too.

The end result is heartburn because the stomach's emptying is reduced. Your body slows down because your body is trying to work through the garbage you just ate. Intuitively, your body slows the digestive processes down, too, which relaxes the upper stomach valve, causing it to open and enter your esophagus, where you will feel a burning sensation. This burning in your esophagus is heartburn. It can even result in an off-taste in your mouth.

Heartburn is a condition that occurs once a week or less. If it happens twice a week or more, it is considered a disorder called gastroesophageal reflux disease (GERD). GERD could also be just a red flag that your diet is bad way too often or you are missing digestive compounds. GERD is a chronic condition that causes long-term damage to the esophagus if not managed.

It's important to keep in mind the severity of your condition. For example, If you have moderate to severe GERD, you really need to seek the help of your doctor or healthcare practitioner. Preferably, see one that can have a conversation about food too and has experience understanding gut health. I suggest seeing a functional medicine doctor or a functional nutritionist.

Advisory: When You Should Seek Medical Advice

Remember, heartburn is a condition that everyone experiences from time to time. While not as serious as GERD, letting it continue unchecked can lead to GERD. You should nip heartburn in the bud by fixing your diet and adding healing supplements. Regular experiencing heartburn and indigestion can also indicate other non-gut-related diseases, so always see your medical practitioner for advice.

Not surprisingly, heartburn will almost always happen due to what you eat. Much more rarely, it is caused by high stomach acid, contrary to popular opinion. But it can be caused by stomach infections too, usually an infection called H. pylori. Infections, by the way, are also related to poor eating patterns.

Personally, I don't have **GERD**, but I do get acid reflux occasionally if I eat gluten, some kinds of dairy products, alcohol, or spicy foods without proper nutritional supplements. I'm among the ranks of most people in this regard. Remember that heartburn is usually triggered by general overindulgence in fried foods, spicy foods, food intolerances, and alcohol, to name a few.

Standard Heartburn Treatment Misses the Mark

Almost no one lives their lives entirely free from heartburn or acid reflux. But it is rarely due to too much acid. However, conventional medications for acid reflux are called proton pump inhibitors (PPIs) or antacids. These medications may help block or reduce acid production, but they often don't really address the underlying causes of the condition. Sadly, they are a conventional band aid for what is almost always an underlying food problem or nutritional problem that can be fixed naturally.

Very importantly, conventional medicines for heartburn and GERD are meant to only be for short-term use because they wreak havoc on long-term health. PPIs in the long term include an increased risk of bone fractures, dementia, infections, heart disease, heart failure, and more. Low stomach acid, ironically, is even actually now recognized as a cause of reflux. Sadly, these PPIs change the chemistry of the digestive tract, making the gut environment inhospitable to healthy bacteria. This is shown repeatedly in the most recent research.[154] [155] PPIs can do this in a very short time, as little as a month.

What we don't know is whether or not someone's gut environment ever returns to normal after stopping medication use. And the whole digestive system suffers when too little acid is caused by medications. This is why some people feel better using natural approaches for heartburn, such as apple cider vinegar (see page 74) or betaine HCL (see page 163). The acid, interestingly, can help their reflux symptoms in many cases.

Remember, at the root of reflux are often poor diets and ultra-processed foods. For this reason, the first line of treatment for acid reflux is addressing your diet and supplementing your diet to rejuvenate your digestive tract.

How Stomach Acid Is Critical for Digestive Health

The natural pH of the stomach is very acidic, around 1–2 pH, and this low pH is for many good reasons. By the way, your stomach acid is much more acidic than lemon juice. A normal stomach produces several quarts of gastric fluid daily, most of which is acid. Stomach acid, or hydrochloric acid, is required for overall health. If you are low in stomach acid, the condition is called hypochlorhydria. This disorder can create many health issues, primarily due to the lack of nutrients related to poor absorption.

The stomach's acidity helps the body to kill unwanted germs and bacteria,

---

[154] Imhann F, Bonder M, et al. Proton pump inhibitors affect the gut microbiome. *Gut.* 2016 May;65(5):740–8.

Macke L, Schulz C, e t al. Systematic review: the effects of proton pump inhibitors on the microbiome of the digestive tract-evidence from next-generation sequencing studies. *Aliment Pharmacol Ther.* 2020 Mar;51(5):505–26.

[155] Cheng J, Ouwehand A. Gastroesophageal reflux disease and probiotics: a systematic review. *Nutrients.* 2020 Jan 2;12(1):132.

stimulates the intestines and pancreas to make digestive enzymes, helps break down proteins so they can be absorbed, helps prevent foodborne illness, helps vitamin B12 absorb, and helps most major minerals absorb. These minerals include calcium, iron, and magnesium, to name a few. Fascinatingly, stomach acid is even required to help keep the stomach contents from flowing into the esophagus.

Stomach acid is also required in the stomach to trigger the opening of the stomach contents into the intestines. This helps to keep food from flowing back into the esophagus. Some cases of "acid reflux" are actually caused by low stomach acid, as mentioned previously.

In summary, stomach acid plays a critical role in getting the nutrients you need from food by helping to stimulate enzymes and breaking down foods for absorption. In other words, you don't want to be without stomach acid. Even people with acidic reflux need stomach acid to properly absorb their food.

Causes and Symptoms of Low Stomach Acid

Some common causes and factors related to low levels of stomach acid are stress, H. pylori infections, antacids, PPIs, imbalanced diets, stomach surgeries, autoimmune conditions, small intestinal bacterial overgrowth (SIBO), vegan or vegetarian diets, diets low in vitamins and minerals, and aging. Zinc and most essential vitamins (see page 100) also help the stomach to make hydrochloric acid. For this reason, imbalanced diets or restrictive diets that are low in absorbable nutrients can cause low stomach acid.

As you can see, there are many causes of low stomach acid, so it is easy to go undiagnosed. So, you can next learn about the symptoms of low stomach acid to see if you may be suffering from this condition.

Symptoms of low stomach acid range from digestive complaints to infections, allergies, and hair loss. In other words, low stomach acid, also known as hypochlorhydria, can affect your whole body. Often, people may mistakenly feel like their stomach acid levels are too high when they are actually too low.

Some commonly reported symptoms of too little stomach acid are bloating, diarrhea, trouble digesting meat, bad breath, increased food allergies, acid reflux, gas, undigested foods in your bowel movements, nausea from vitamin supplements, nutrient deficiencies, hair loss in women, brittle nails, yeast infections, and mood swings.

Your stomach acid helps to break your food down and kill unwanted germs. When you lack stomach acid, food doesn't digest well, so the whole body becomes deprived of nutrients, and bacteria levels get out of balance.

Did You Know . . . About the Baking Soda Test

The only way to know if you have low or high stomach acid levels is to check your pH. You can ask your doctor, but this test is done with a pH probe, which is a bit invasive. For this reason, it is not done frequently. It is also possible to do a simple test at home. Keep in mind this test is only accurate at the moment. Your stomach pH can vary depending on when you last ate food, the timing of the day, etc. But it's much easier than a stomach probe, and it's also safe to try as long as you only use it occasionally.

- First thing in the morning, before food, drinking, or brushing, mix ¼ teaspoon of baking soda into 4 oz of warm water.
- Drink this mixture and immediately set a timer to see how long it takes to burp.
- You should belch fairly quickly afterward if your stomach makes acid.
- If it takes you more than 3−5 minutes to burp, you are likely not making enough stomach acid. This is because baking soda is alkaline, and when it mixes with hydrochloric acid in the stomach, it creates bubbles that rise. In a healthy stomach, these bubbles will form quite quickly.

While this does not provide a diagnosis of low stomach acid, it can help you have a conversation with your healthcare provider about the appropriate tests and treatments for you.

Note: Baking soda is also used to neutralize stomach acid, which can make your stomach feel off or nauseated for a bit. It does for me.

Easy Fixes Heartburn Relief

Eating a well-balanced diet may help balance stomach acid production naturally over time and can also help resolve nutritional issues that are causing your heartburn. But, if you have been eating the wrong foods for a long time or have suffered from heartburn for a long time, you will get better more quickly by supplementing vitamins and minerals, digestive enzyme supplements, probiotics, and holistic herbs.

Foods that are whole and unprocessed are your best bets for easing heartburn. And a super simple trick is to chew your food well and eat slowly. As a rule, avoid packaged foods, fried foods, and high-sugar foods and beverages. It is also extremely important to figure out if you are sensitive to certain foods. Common ones are wheat, dairy, soy, corn, nightshade foods (i.e., tomatoes, potatos, peppers, and eggplant), citrus, and more. Alcohol and caffeinated beverages are also very common acid reflux triggers. Although identifying these food sensitivities is beyond the scope of this book, there are many books out there that can be helpful, including my books, *The Whole Body Guide to Gut Health* and *The Elimination Diet Journal*.

Fermented Foods

By far, one of the best digestive aids for heartburn is sauerkraut. Time and time again, my clients swear that it is one of the most important things they have added to their diet to feel better from heartburn or other digestive conditions. While raw sauerkraut is mostly used as a natural probiotic, it makes sense that it can help with low stomach acid because it provides a natural level of acid for the stomach too. It also provides a natural source of digestive enzymes.

Apple Cider Vinegar

This also helps to acidify the stomach, and it is a source of beneficial probiotics. This is true if you buy the apple cider vinegar "with the mother." Honestly, there is no research to back that apple cider vinegar truly helps with low stomach acid, but logic contends that it does. Countless people swear by this remedy for an upset stomach and for improving overall digestive function.

Be sure to dilute apple cider vinegar with water or extra virgin olive oil. A common practice is to drink 16 oz of water with 2 tablespoons of apple cider vinegar daily and drink it with your main meal. Mixing it with honey is also common practice; honey is a good stomach tonic because it contains natural prebiotics. You can also use apple cider vinegar capsules but don't exceed the recommended dose on the label, and make sure to take it with water as well.

Herbs and Spices

Using culinary herbs and spices, sometimes called bitters, like fenugreek, dandelion root, fennel seed, cardamom, chamomile, yarrow, mint, and caraway is also a smart idea if you struggle with heartburn. A good way to use these is to make herbal tea infusions by simply steeping these herbs in water.

Did You Know . . . Stress and Heartburn Are Related

Emotional stress can trigger many imbalances in the body, including heartburn. I know many patients who say that stress can be the number one cause of their acid reflux and heartburn symptoms. While this may be true, one of the main contributors to daily stress is an imbalanced diet and lack of key nutrients.

Focusing on stress management is an important part of all aspects of health, so take time in your day to de-stress, meditate, and relax. Also, fixing your diet and nutrition can help with your stress, so the benefits of supplements and diet are circular.

Supplements to Heal Low Stomach Acid

If your low stomach acid is due to medications, please check with your doctor to find the best way to help manage this. Otherwise, natural remedies for low stomach acid and/or heartburn include probiotics, fermented foods, betaine HCL, digestive enzymes, bovine colostrum, vitamins and minerals, ginger, marshmallow root, slippery elm, and diet changes as described earlier.

Let's delve into each of these more and how they can help your low stomach acid levels and your indigestion and heartburn maladies.

Probiotics

Probiotics were traditionally used to treat lower GI symptoms, but research shows that certain beneficial bacteria may help with many aspects of upper digestive health, including reflux and heartburn.[156] Probiotic strains are very well tolerated and improve various reflux and other gut symptoms. It is important to note that the studies first ruled out helicobacter pylori (H. pylori) infections, which can be a source of acid reflux. To date, eight major strains of probiotics have been studied, and by balancing out the gut microbiome, probiotics can have far-reaching effects.

One study investigating reflux used probiotics as an add-on to proton pump inhibitors (PPIs), the standard treatment for GERD-related symptoms. It demonstrated superior benefits to using conventional PPI treatment alone.[157] But even those that only experience occasional stomach pain can benefit gastric benefits of probiotics too. For example, a follow-up study of *Bifidobacterium bifidum* fermented milk in healthy adults found that this

[156] Sun Q, Wang H, et al. Beneficial effect of probiotics supplements in reflux esophagitis treated with esomeprazole: a randomized controlled trial. World J Gastroenterol. 2019 May 7;25(17):2110–21.

[157] Cheng J, Ouwehand A. Gastroesophageal reflux disease and probiotics: a systematic review. *Nutrients.* 2020 Jan 2;12(1):132.

supplement reduced stomach pain and increased overall post-meal comfort compared to a placebo.[158]

A perk of using *Lactobacillus gasseri* yogurt is that it may reduce abdominal fat by as much as 8–9 percent compared to conventional yogurt over twelve weeks. [159] *Lactobacillus gasseri* also reduced waist circumference and abdominal fat, according to another study, especially when using a higher dose (10 billion CFU). [160] At this point in time, however, it isn't possible to find this type of yogurt, but you can make your own by buying *Lactobacillus gasseri* supplements and fermenting your own yogurt with it.

Here is a summary of how each probiotic strain works. When choosing a probiotic supplement for heartburn, choose one with more than one of these strains.

- Bifidobacterium lactis—increases stomach emptying and speeds up intestinal movement time. Eight of nine belly symptoms improved in research studies.[161]
- Bacillus subtilis—decreases SIBO and many GI symptoms, including indigestion. This is found in many soil-based probiotic supplements.[162]
- Lactobacillus gasseri—may help to eliminate heartburn and reflux

---

[158] Kadooka Y, Sato M, et al. Effect of Lactobacillus gasseri SBT2055 in fermented milk on abdominal adiposity in adults in a randomised controlled trial. *Br J Nutr.* 2013 Nov 14;110(9):1696–703.

[159] Urita Y, Goto M, et al. Continuous consumption of fermented milk containing Bifidobacterium bifidum YIT 10347 improves gastrointestinal and psychological symptoms in patients with functional gastrointestinal disorders. Biosci Microbiota Food Health. 2015;34(2):37–44.

[160] Kim J, Yun J, et al. Lactobacillus gasseri BNR17 supplementation reduces the visceral fat accumulation and waist circumference in obese adults: a randomized, double-blind, placebo-controlled trial. *J Med Food.* 2018 May;21(5):454–61.

[161] Waller P, Gopal P, et al. Dose-response effect of Bifidobacterium lactis HN019 on whole gut transit time and functional gastrointestinal symptoms in adults. *Scand J Gastroenterol.* 2011 Sep;46(9):1057–64.

[162] Kadooka Y, Sato M, et al. Effect of Lactobacillus gasseri SBT2055 in fermented milk on abdominal adiposity in adults in a randomised controlled trial. *Br J Nutr.* 2013 Nov 14;110(9):1696–703.

symptoms as well as reduce abdominal fat and waist circumference.[163]
- *Bifidobacterium bifidum*—may decrease abdominal pain, diarrhea, and constipation.[164]
- *Lactobacillus reuteri*—may reduce colic, reduce vomiting, and increase bowel movement frequency which can ultimately help reduce heartburn. Also decreases abdominal pain, distention, nausea, and vomiting.[165] [166]
- *Lactobacillus rhamnosus GG*—decreased abdominal pain, distention (a cause of heartburn), nausea, and vomiting.[167]
- *Saccharomyces boulardii*—along with L. reuteri, this strain may help reduce colic and vomiting and alleviate constipation which can be a root cause of heartburn.[168]
- *E. faecium*—could be helpful for many aspects of GI health, but not currently available commercially yet.[169]

Probiotics may help combat a root cause of acid reflux, too—H. pylori

[163] Kim J, Yun J, et al. Lactobacillus gasseri BNR17 supplementation reduces the visceral fat accumulation and waist circumference in obese adults: a randomized, double-blind, placebo-controlled trial. *J Med Food.* 2018 May;21(5):454–61.

[164] Urita Y, Goto M, et al. Continuous consumption of fermented milk containing Bifidobacterium bifidum YIT 10347 improves gastrointestinal and psychological symptoms in patients with functional gastrointestinal disorders. *Biosci Microbiota Food Health.* 2015;34(2):37–44.

[165] Indrio F, Riezzo G, et al. Lactobacillus reuteri accelerates gastric emptying and improves regurgitation in infants. *Eur J Clin Invest.* 2011 Apr;41(4):417–22.

[166] Indrio F, Di Mauro A, et al. Prophylactic use of a probiotic in the prevention of colic, regurgitation, and functional constipation: a randomized clinical trial. *JAMA Pediatr.* 2014 Mar;168(3):228–33.

[167] Ianiro G, Pizzoferrato M, et al. Effect of an extra-virgin olive oil enriched with probiotics or antioxidants on functional dyspepsia: a pilot study. *Eur Rev Med Pharmacol Sci.* 2013;17(15):2085–90. PMID: 23884830.

[168] Kelesidis T, Pothoulakis C. Efficacy and safety of the probiotic Saccharomyces boulardii for the prevention and therapy of gastrointestinal disorders. *Therap Adv Gastroenterol.* 2012 Mar;5(2):111–25.

[169] Zhou X, Willems R, et al. Enterococcus faecium: from microbiological insights to practical recommendations for infection control and diagnostics. *Antimicrob Resist Infect Control.* 2020 Aug 10;9(1):130.

infections. For example, one study found that using the *Bifidobacterium infantis* plus conventional antibiotics was better than treatment alone in a study of people with helicobacter pylori infections.[170] The antibiotics-only treatment eradicated H.Pylori at 69 percent. In comparison, pre-treatment with the probiotic *Bifidobacterium infantis* for two weeks and during antibiotic treatment led to a 91 percent eradication of H. pylori. Using fermented yogurts that are rich in probiotics reduces H. pylori infections as well, according to other research. [171]

Betaine HCL

Betaine HCL is a dietary supplement that helps to acidify the stomach. As you may recall, the root cause of heartburn can be too little acid instead of too much, so many people find relief when they take betaine HCL. Just make sure to take the capsules right before eating. Using betaine HCL helps many people with their GI reflux symptoms and even gallbladder issues, too, according to reviews.

Bear in mind most of these reports are not yet proven out in research, so try them with caution and always discuss adding betaine HCL with your healthcare provider. Still, they are safe to try for most people, and there are thousands of positive reviews of how betaine HCL improves heartburn symptoms. Of note, there is another kind of betaine supplement called TMG (trimethylglycine) which may have calming effects, so it also may help with gut health. It does not acidify the stomach, however.

---

[170] Dajani A, Abu Hammour A, et al. Do probiotics improve eradication response to Helicobacter pylori on standard triple or sequential therapy? *Saudi J Gastroenterol.* 2013 May-Jun;19(3):113–20.

[171] Sachdeva A, Nagpal J. Effect of fermented milk-based probiotic preparations on Helicobacter pylori eradication: a systematic review and meta-analysis of randomized-controlled trials. *Eur J Gastroenterol Hepatol.* 2009 Jan;21(1):45–53.

Digestive Enzymes

Digestive enzymes' roles are to break down your foods so that you can absorb them, so as you can imagine, they also play a role in preventing heartburn. These enzymes are made all throughout the upper digestive tract, starting in your mouth. In your stomach, pepsin enzymes are made to help your body break down protein and help you digest vitamin B12. And stomach acid helps to activate all of the enzymes, including pepsin, that your GI tract makes.

Chronic digestive disorders cause inflammation in the gut lining, where most digestive enzymes are made. So when you have inflammation in your gut, the ability to make enzymes diminishes. As you might imagine, this inflammatory process is a problem for almost everyone eating a Western diet.

Digestive enzymes simply help you digest foods better, making the whole eating experience more pleasant and resulting in less heartburn. It is my go-to for helping my stomach and esophagus tolerate spicy foods. The bonus is that you will likely get more nutrition to absorb from your foods and have less gas and bloating. After all, when you have enough enzymes, your digestive tract can do the job that it is intended to do.

As your digestive tract begins doing what it should: digest foods, you also may find that spicy or acidic food are not really the issue at all for reflux. It's indigestion! When you use a broad-spectrum digestive enzyme, foods get broken down more readily, so easing gas and bloating and may reduce acid reflux. Supplemental enzymes likely help food move along so it doesn't linger in the stomach long enough to create acid reflux.

The stomach has a valve called a lower esophageal sphincter. This valve makes it so foods can empty into the small intestine for digestion. If you have too little stomach acid or not enough enzymes, this sphincter won't allow foods to empty properly. Thus, a lack of enzymes may, in fact, be the root of your acid reflux, according to research. [172] [173]

The first thing to know when purchasing digestive enzyme supplements is that they vary wildly. Some have one type of enzyme, such as Lactaid, which contains lactase to help digest milk. Other broad-spectrum enzymes help digest various foods and break down difficult-to-digest compounds. Broad spectrum enzymes will include amylase, protease, lipase, lactase, sucrase, alpha-amylase, maltase, cellulase, hemicellulase, pectinase, phytase, alpha-galactosidase, and endopeptidase.

A broad-spectrum enzyme supplement will be inherently better for most aspects of digestive function than single-enzyme supplements. In other words, skip the Beano and Lactaid, and get a supplement that can help you break down all the fibers, starches, fats, and proteins, as well as lactose, in your diet. Broad-spectrum enzymes help make more digestible compounds such as amino acids, short-chain fatty acids, and simple carbohydrates that can cross the gut barrier wall. Refer back to Chapter 7 for more information about digestive enzymes.

Bovine Colostrum

Bovine colostrum is great for overall health and is one of many tools that may help heal your stomach lining from ongoing reflux (see Chapter 5, page 60). Remember, though, that colostrum is derived from dairy, so if you are allergic to milk products, you should avoid colostrum. However, if you are lactose intolerant, you should be fine taking colostrum because it is very low in lactose. Start with a teaspoon daily and work your way up to taking a tablespoon daily for overall stomach and immune health.

---

[172] Bardhan K, Strugala V, Dettmar P. Reflux revisited: Advancing the role of pepsin. *Int J Otolaryngol.* 2012;2012:646901.

[173] Majeed M, Majeed S, Nagabhushanam K, et al. Evaluation of the safety and efficacy of a multienzyme complex in patients with functional dyspepsia: A randomized, double-blind, placebo-controlled study. *Journal of Medicinal Food.* Nov 2018.1120–8.

Vitamins and Minerals

If you have struggled with heartburn, you may not have considered the role of vitamins and minerals in its causes and treatment. But you can think of it like this: nutrients are the building blocks for everything in your body, including the structure of your stomach, its lining, its acid balance, and its enzymes.

When you have low vitamin or mineral levels, your stomach is more vulnerable to infections, inflammation, indigestion, reflux, disease, and ulceration. And if you are among the ranks of most people, you are likely low in at least one or more nutrients. A good example is that lacking zinc may contribute to stomach acid ulcers, and supplemental zinc may help reduce their risk. Zinc carnosine may be especially protective for helping heal the stomach lining.

If you are looking for a good vitamin and mineral supplement, I recommend choosing all-natural brands. One of the best ways to naturally get more vitamins and minerals is to supplement with grass-finished beef liver capsules. After all, liver organ meat is the most concentrated source of nutrients on the planet. You can also get all-natural multivitamins with minerals; see page 304 for my recommended brands. Just take your multivitamin and mineral supplements, including zinc, with food.

Other Heartburn Therapies

There are several other herbal therapies for heartburn and indigestion, including:

- Marshmallow root: See Chapter 7
- Ginger root: See Chapter 7
- Licorice root: For short-term use unless you use deglycyrrhizinated licorice. Also, do not take it with high blood pressure unless it is deglycyrrhizinated licorice.
- Slippery elm: See Chapter 7

- Aloe vera: See Chapter 7
- Iberogast: See Chapter 7
- Fennel seeds: Simply chew ¼ teaspoon of seeds or make tea with these seeds as needed.
- Lemon zest: Take 1 g (a quarter teaspoon) daily to see if it helps your stomach distress.
- Lemon balm: It makes a great tea, but it is also available in tincture form. Take 1 dropperful up to five times a day.
- Mint: Helps to reduce dyspepsia and is often used in gel caps. Typically, 1 gel cap is all you need. You can also easily make mint tea if you wish.
- Triphala: Take 1–2 capsules a day.

As a general rule, I suggest following the dosing recommendations in Chapter 7 or following the label instructions. Also, in the next paragraphs I suggest dosing where it may vary from the common label directions.

Marshmallow root: Provides a protective coating of mucilage to the stomach, so many people feel soothed when they use marshmallow root. It is commonly used to help heal gastric ulcers as well.

Licorice root: A common stomach remedy and helpful for heartburn too. Remember that it is meant for short-term use unless you use deglycyrrhizinated licorice. Also, do not take licorice root if you have high blood pressure unless it is deglycyrrhizinated licorice.

Slippery elm: Similar to marshmallow root because it provides a protective coat for the stomach.

Aloe vera: Clinically shown to help reduce heartburn symptoms because it is rich in antioxidants. However, it can potentially increase diarrhea symptoms if it contains parts of the skin. Nature's Way or Global Healing has reputable aloe vera supplements.

Iberogast: A branded herbal supplement with peppermint, licorice root, and milk thistle. Several studies have shown that this herbal combination effectively relieves heartburn and GERD.

Fennel seeds: Great for reducing gas and bloating associated with indigestion by helping the stomach empty more easily. Simply chew on ¼ teaspoon of seeds or make tea with these seeds as needed.

Lemon zest (not lemon juice): This helps to increase the mucus production of the stomach, so it may help alleviate heartburn symptoms. You can use 1 g of lemon zest (1 quarter teaspoon) daily to see if it helps your stomach distress.

Lemon balm: A relaxing herb that can help settle the stomach because of this. It makes a great tea, but it is also available in tincture form. Take 1 dropperful up to 5 times a day.

Mint: Helps to reduce dyspepsia for many people and is often used in gel caps. Typically, 1 gel cap is all you need. You can also easily make fresh mint tea.

Triphala. Reduces heartburn and indigestion by reducing gas and bloating for some people. Typically 1–2 capsules are used.

Fish Oil and Cod Liver Oil

Fish oil and cod liver oil are both rich in omega-3 fats that help dampen inflammation. New research even shows that these healthy fats act as prebiotics in the gut. [174] This means that they help probiotics survive and thrive in the digestive tract. Early research shows that they may reduce reflux and increase antioxidants in the stomach.[175] Cod liver oil is preferred over fish oil for gut health because it is a natural source of healing vitamin A, and it also is easier to absorb.

Melatonin

Melatonin is naturally made in the body as a sleep hormone, but it's also found in foods and can be a healthy supplement for overall health. One of its

---

[174] Vijay A, Astbury S, et al. The prebiotic effects of omega-3 fatty acid supplementation: A six-week randomised intervention trial. *Gut Microbes.* 2021 Jan-Dec;13(1):1–11.

[175] Zhuang Z, Xie J, et al. The effect of n-3/n-6 polyunsaturated fatty acids on acute reflux esophagitis in rats. *Lipids Health Dis.* 2016 Oct 4;15(1):172.

fascinating benefits is that it may reduce the incidences of heartburn. Low levels of melatonin are linked to an increased risk of getting heartburn as well. It also serves as an antioxidant in the body. Taking melatonin at low doses, around 3–5 mg daily, is safe for most people. However, the occasional person can experience nightmares from taking it.

Activated Charcoal

Using activated charcoal for heartburn may seem unusual, but natural practitioners for thousands of years have turned to charcoal for its many digestive benefits. Some research even shows that it helps reduce heartburn and dyspepsia.[176] With an absorptive area of 1000 m^2 per serving, activated charcoal can adsorb lots of unwanted compounds and reduce gas buildup in the stomach, which contributes to the feelings of reflux.

Often made from coconut husks, this natural compound is actually very safe. In my experience, activated charcoal is nice to have on hand for an occasional overindulgence of food, and it really works to alleviate belly distress. But it is only meant to be used occasionally because it may bind nutrients in the gut. When using activated charcoal, follow the label instructions, and do not use this remedy if you are constipated.

Cannabis

Cannabidiol, or CBD, is a natural compound in hemp and cannabis. This compound may help many aspects of digestive function and may even help reduce the chances of heartburn. Research shows that there are cannabinoid receptors in the esophagus. Both CBD and THC may serve as anti-inflammatory compounds in the upper digestive tract and improve both

---

[176] Coffin B, Bortolloti C, et al. Efficacy of a simethicone, activated charcoal and magnesium oxide combination (CarbosymagB®) in functional dyspepsia: Results of a general practice-based randomized trial. *Clin. Res. Hepatol. Gastroenterol.* 2011;35:494–9.

stomach and esophagus function. [177]

However, only certain US states have legalized full-spectrum cannabis. In states where it is legal, using edibles with high THC can have unwanted side effects for people new to these compounds if they don't use them slowly and carefully. That said, many people find CBD and THC helpful for reducing feelings of anxiety, and this, in turn, may reduce heartburn indirectly. Just make sure to start low and slow when using any cannabis products to help reduce the chances of any side effects.

Case Study: Easing Reflux the Natural Way

Acid reflux and indigestion plagued Don for most of his life. He was frustrated because taking his omeprazole prescription only made him feel more tired while minimally alleviating his gut symptoms. He loved fried foods and bread but realized that these were his biggest food triggers, so he decided to eliminate them upon my advice. He began eating more whole foods that weren't in packages too. He also avoided eating at bedtime and began chewing his food more thoroughly. These helped his symptoms, but he still had frequent breakthrough heartburn symptoms.

He agreed to try taking broad-spectrum natural vitamins and minerals daily, betaine HCL, taking a broad-spectrum digestive enzyme with meals, a daily probiotic, and DGL licorice. Almost immediately, his heartburn symptoms disappeared entirely. He is pleased that his stomach problems are gone; he has more energy and doesn't have brain fog anymore at work. He was also able to eliminate the need for taking omeprazole. A few weeks in, he was able to stop taking DGL licorice and betaine HCL but wanted to keep taking the rest of the supplements, including the digestive enzymes, probiotics, and vitamins, because of his much-improved energy and vitality.

---

[177] Gotfried J, Kataria R, et al. Review: The role of cannabinoids on esophageal function—what we know thus far. *Cannabis Cannabinoid Res.* 2017 Oct 1;2(1):252–8.

10

Chapter 10

Nausea: Helpful Remedies

If you have ever felt nauseous, you probably know it can come on out of the blue and be from so many causes that it can seem extremely daunting. However, there are some supplements that you may not be aware of that can help reduce the severity of nausea safely.

Before we get into possible supplements and dietary strategies for each type of nausea, you should know the root causes so nausea can be mitigated before it becomes unmanageable. However, some supplements can cause nausea if not taken correctly, too, so throughout this book, I always make recommendations to ease this. You should also know when to seek help, which will be reviewed.

Common Triggers

There are many possible causes of nausea; just about any health issue can cause it. Additionally, a good majority of prescription medications can lead to it. But you should know that nausea often has an important role in the body: it tells you something is wrong, and you should do something differently to change the triggers. After all, nausea can even be triggered by something as simple as wearing too-tight pants, and that is certainly an easy fix.

Let's start with other easy fixes for nausea. Almost any prescription medication can cause nausea, and usually, the easiest way to fix this is to avoid taking the medication on an empty stomach. Or, you could have a conversation with your provider about minimizing your need for prescription medications in the first place. Having said that, some medications like narcotics medications post-surgery, and chemotherapy don't have easy fixes (and taking anti-nausea drugs and PPIs given for nausea can damage the gut). This can require a lot of healing time with nutrients and supplements due to the side effects of the medications themselves. Even so, some supplements can help ease nausea with these medicines, as we will review.

Also, discuss with your healthcare provider if any lifestyle adjustments can be employed before surgery. For example, could herbal therapies that help your uterine issues be used so you don't have to have a hysterectomy. Far too many times, I meet people who have surgeries, and then their gut issues never go back to normal, so avoiding surgeries when possible is best. A second opinion with a functional medicine doctor is a good idea in many cases. My provider did this for me, and I will be forever grateful.

Even natural drugs like coffee, tea, and caffeine or other stimulants are also very common triggers of nausea, so the obvious fix is to minimize your intake. Taking vitamin supplements and even some natural supplements like glutamine can definitely trigger nausea because they are so concentrated. The easiest fix is to choose natural ones, as described in Chapter 6, and to make sure to start at low doses or to take them with food. The supplements will absorb better, and you will feel better, too, if you do this.

If you have diabetes, preventing the underlying causes of nausea means very tight control of blood glucose management so your stomach isn't damaged by long-term elevated blood sugars. This is beyond the scope of this book, but many people find that if they start early on a lower carbohydrate diet, they can prevent many of the issues associated with type 2 diabetes. And some conditions, like severe kidney disease, can cause nausea, and the only way that this can be treated is through medical management.

Advisory: When to Seek Help

While natural remedies can help many types of temporary nausea, feeling nauseated can be a sign of a serious medical condition, so there are times when nausea becomes an urgent condition. For example, nausea that lasts for extended periods needs to be worked up with a healthcare provider. If you have been vomiting for over two days, you should see your doctor. Or, if you have had periodic nausea and vomiting for longer than a month or so, you should also seek medical advice.

Natural Remedies for Nausea

From pregnancy to motion sickness, digestive issues, infections, stress, and food intolerances, all can cause nausea. Still, all of these often have some natural supplement strategies to help with these symptoms of nausea.

Overcoming Vitamin and Mineral Deficiency

It may actually come as a surprise that a good quality vitamin and mineral can help with nausea. For example, a lack of thiamine, vitamin B6, or niacin, to name a few, can cause nausea, as reviewed in Chapter 10. So repletion of these nutrients can help alleviate nausea for some people. Just make sure to take high-quality vitamins and minerals with food. However, the wrong forms can cause nausea, such as synthetic ones.

Remedies for Gas and Bloating

Excessive abdominal gas and bloating aren't benign conditions; far from it. Having a bloated belly can lead to feelings of nausea and are a sign that your diet is out of balance, your gut is out of balance, or both.

Gas bubbles in the stomach are most prone to leading to nausea. Some people swallow a lot of air when they are chewing, and this can cause feelings of nausea. Try to eat slowly and avoid gulping air. Additionally, stomach emptying can be impaired by a diet filled with processed foods, causing gas, bloating, and nausea.

A few simple and safe remedies to alleviate nausea related to gas and bloating include broad-spectrum digestive enzymes (see Chapter 6) and ginger, peppermint, caraway, fennel, and cardamom (see Chapter 7). Additionally, having some activated charcoal on hand can be a pretty quick remedy to help reduce gas symptoms for occasional nausea caused by gas and bloating. The nice thing is that you can try one or more of these safely simultaneously.

Specifically:

Digestive Enzymes: Take 1 capsule or as directed by the supplement label.

Ginger: I recommend having crystallized ginger or ginger tea every 15 minutes until symptoms subside.

Peppermint: Keep some peppermint gel caps handy and take one as needed. Or drink a cup of peppermint tea.

Caraway or fennel: Chew up ⅛ teaspoon of whole caraway or fennel seeds to alleviate nausea caused by gas.

Cardamom: Chew 1 cardamom pod or make tea out of 1 teaspoon of cardamom pods.

Activated charcoal: Follow package directions for the recommended dose, usually 1–2 capsules for occasional nausea.

Motion Sickness

I wish that I could give you an extensive list of remedies, but there are only a few that seem to help. Taking ginger capsules an hour before your trip can be very helpful because they help speed up recovery from motion. Additionally, using peppermint in gel caps can help. I also find that keeping my nasal and sinus passages clear helps with a natural sinus spray containing herbs (see page 309 for recommendations). It will initially burn the nostrils, but it's well worth it. There is no shame in taking Dramamine or Bonine on top of these, either.

Other than that, eating well the day before and the day of, staying well-hydrated, and hoping for a good trip can help. I also recommend trying

clinical hypnotherapy or **tapping techniques** to ease the anxiety associated with flying if you tend to get sick.

Food Intolerances

Conventional practitioners can lead you to believe that food intolerances, sensitivities, and allergies are rare when nothing is further from the truth. Most people I meet these days have one or more of the above. Whatever the reason for the rise in sensitivities, it is here to stay, it seems. While there are some differences between food sensitivities and intolerances, the net result is often the same; gut misery.

However, many people suffer in silence for years, waiting for their GI doc to test them, and it never gets done. This is because the only true gold standard is an elimination diet, and many people shy away from doing these (even though they aren't that bad!) There are lots of books that help do these. They vary in style, including books like The Wahls Protocol by Dr. Terry Wahls, my book *The Whole Body Guide to Gut Health*, *The Microbiome Connection* (low fermentation diet) by Dr. Mark Pimentel, Low FODMAPS cookbooks, **Paleo** diet books, and more.

If you suspect you are sensitive or intolerant and it is causing nausea, the most effective way to alleviate this is to avoid or limit the offending food. However, I live in the real world and know this isn't always possible. For example, I'm sensitive to gluten but occasionally indulge in it. I use a good broad-spectrum digestive enzyme along with activated charcoal when I do decide it's worth the risk of indulging. I only indulge for one day and return to my usual gluten-free diet, or my gut goes into a tailspin.

For mild food intolerances, I recommend eating digestive enzymes with these foods, and you can review how to get the best kinds in Chapter 7. However, food sensitivities and allergies are more serious because they cause the whole body to be inflamed. If your joints hurt, your skin breaks out, your brain is foggy, or worse, due to an offending food, it is best to take the elimination of this food more seriously. Refer to Chapter 17 on how to deal with food intolerances, sensitivities, and allergies.

That said, some supplements may help your gut become more tolerant over time, but there's really no way to know if they will work for sure. It's certainly worth a try because they are healthy anyways. For many people, adding in bovine colostrum or IGG supplements helps heal their gut well enough that they can tolerate more foods. Or adding organ meat supplements like intestines may also be helpful. Adding these supplements can take several months to help reduce food intolerances and sensitivities.

Dysbiosis

Dysbiosis is an imbalance in the natural bacteria in the gut. This condition can result in many symptoms, including nausea and indigestion. A good example of this is SIBO and IBS. While diet and supplements may not always be enough to fix these conditions alone, they often can be standalone therapy because the imbalance in the diet is usually where dysbiosis begins. Some signs of dysbiosis can include a white coating on the tongue or abnormal color to your tongue, bad breath, upper abdominal pain, heartburn, constipation, diarrhea, and of course, nausea.

A good starting place is to minimize or avoid alcohol, sugary foods and drinks, and any unnecessary prescriptions for antibiotics. Eat a good amount of protein, around 30 g per meal or more, to help provide the building blocks of healthy cells in the gut. Additionally, include lots of healthy fats like extra virgin olive oil, avocados, coconut oil, and nuts while skipping processed foods. It is also a good idea to limit or avoid legumes and many grains while healing.

Some helpful supplements for nausea caused by dysbiosis include:

MCT oil: This can be a helpful addition, especially if dysbiosis occurs in the small intestine. Start slowly with 1 teaspoon daily and SLOWLY sip it with a beverage.

Probiotics: The best probiotics for dysbiosis often are spore-based ones.

Digestive enzymes: These are a cornerstone to making just about everything work better and can reduce nausea related to dysbiosis.

Bovine colostrum: This healing supplement can help boost your body's immune system and helps scavenge unwanted bacteria. It also helps heal the gut lining. Generally, starting with a teaspoon twice a day and working up to 1 tablespoon twice a day can be very helpful.

Natural multivitamins with minerals: This is a critical step to boost your body's own immune function to fight off unwanted bacteria and fungi.

Ginger: This can be helpful in almost every kind of nausea, including dysbiosis-induced nausea. It speeds up gut motility, making nausea less likely. It also supports the growth of beneficial bacteria while deterring harmful bacteria.

If you have SIBO or candida overgrowth, you may need additional strategies, such as natural antimicrobial therapies. This is best done under the supervision of a well-trained functional medicine doctor or nutritionist.

Stress

Nausea is stressful any way you look at it, but which came first, the chicken or the egg? Stress itself is also nauseating. Managing stress well should be the first recommendation here, and it is. But, due to the gut-brain axis, stress is often rooted in gut imbalances. So we are going in circles, but ultimately, by taking care of your gut and replenishing your nutrient stores, you can reduce stress-induced nausea. Research also shows that stress can make your body depleted of nutrients,[178] so no, diet isn't typically enough to overcome the deficits of stress.

Several stress-reducing supplements can include:

Natural multivitamins with minerals: As reviewed in Chapter 6.

Probiotics: Almost every probiotic strain available today may help reduce the body's stress response and anxiety symptoms, according to research.[179] The best probiotic for stress, then, is one you can afford and tolerate.

---

[178] Vitellio P, Chira A, et al. Probiotics in psychosocial stress and anxiety. a systematic review. *J Gastrointestin Liver Dis.* 2020 Mar 13;29(1):77–83.

[179] Lopresti A. The effects of psychological and environmental stress on micronutrient concentrations in the body: a review of the evidence. *Adv Nutr.* 2020 Jan 1;11(1):103–12.

Tulsi (holy basil): Reduces feelings of stress in the body and even helps boost immune function. Tulsi makes great tea, and I recommend sipping on some daily. This herb is eaten daily by some cultures.

Lavender: This calming herb is very powerful for reducing anxiety and stress in some people. You can buy capsules, as reviewed in Chapter 7. Follow the supplement suggestions for dosing.

Cannabis: For many people, an effective way to cut nausea due to stress is medicinal cannabis. But, be aware that it can be very strong, so using very low doses is recommended. Typically, *Indica* strains are the most calming ones. Be aware that too much can make you nauseated too. Every person has their own threshold, so tread lightly.

Fish oil: Every cell membrane in the body needs omega-3 fats, so if you are low, your body's ability to handle stress is impaired. Just make sure to take fish oil with food so that you don't have any unintended side effects.

Ashwagandha: Functions as an adaptogen, so it helps reduce stress if used regularly. I prefer to get ashwagandha in tea form along with tulsi. Organic India makes a nice tulsi ashwagandha tea you can buy in health food stores or online. Large doses of ashwagandha can cause nausea for some people, so start with a low dose if you take it in capsule form.

Chamomile: This is a surprisingly potent herb for stress relief, and it even soothes an upset stomach. Both tea and capsule forms are good choices to help relieve stress-related nausea.

Lemon balm: This herb is also calming and soothing to the stomach during times of stress. It is often found in relaxing and sleepy tea for this reason.

Indigestion and Heartburn

A common cause of nausea is indigestion, so to relieve it, you can read all about heartburn, indigestion, and remedies for these in Chapter 9. The root cause is usually an imbalance in the diet, so it is best to address this first, such as eliminating processed foods, fried foods, and offending foods like gluten, alcohol, caffeine, soy, or dairy.

Here is a checklist of remedies for nausea related to heartburn and indigestion.

Licorice root: A favorite for nausea relief in this setting. Use either licorice tea or DGL licorice supplements. If you use licorice frequently, read all about it in chapter 7.

Digestive enzymes: Help break down foods that are the root cause of nausea. Taking them after a meal can even help in my experience.

Ginger root: A wonderful digestive aid that is great as tea, crystallized ginger, or ginger capsules.

Fennel: A great digestive aid to relieve many aspects of indigestion, including nausea.

Cardamom: A warming spice that works well for nausea related to dyspepsia and indigestion. Have some cardamom tea, or add some ground cardamom to just about any recipe.

Lemon zest: The antioxidants in lemon zest can calm down nausea due to indigestion, and this is an easy trick because lemon zest can be added to water, tea, and almost any recipe.

Peppermint: Soothing in the case of indigestion and nausea, which always seems to provide relief quite quickly. Using peppermint tea or gel caps is a good option.

Probiotics: As with almost any digestive condition, probiotics can help reduce nausea related to indigestion because these healthy bacteria can help break down foods.

Activated charcoal: This is a safe rescue for occasional nausea associated with indigestion.

Iberogast: A trademark name of an effective herbal blend used to help treat nausea related to indigestion and dyspepsia.

Pregnancy

The time in many people's lives when most women experience some nausea, is during pregnancy—me included. While there are no sure bet fixes, the same rules apply here: avoiding foods that cause gut sensitivities and promoting healthy digestive function and nutrition through natural approaches can help.

Some research-validated and safe tools to help with nausea during pregnancy are:

Probiotics: Reduce nausea and vomiting symptoms during pregnancy, and the probiotic benefits are even passed to the baby. [180]

Prebiotics: These can help promote probiotic growth in the gut and help with bowel regularity. Just be sure to review the prebiotics section in Chapter 8.[181]

P5P: The active and natural form of vitamin B6, and it reduces nausea safely during pregnancy. [182] [183]

Ginger: This is a safe and effective remedy for nausea during pregnancy. Doses of up to 1g per day are safe, or sip fresh ginger tea made with ¼ inch peeled ginger root steeped in hot water.

Peppermint: Drinking peppermint tea or simply inhaling the scent of peppermint can alleviate nausea during pregnancy.[184]

Folate: Taken as 5 MTHF should be used instead of folic acid if you have a gene variant of folate metabolism, which about half of women do. In this case, using a natural prenatal vitamin is best such as Pure Encapsulations Prenatal Nutrients. It contains natural and activated folate, which is easier

---

[180] Martín-Peláez S, Cano-Ibáñez N, et al. The impact of probiotics, prebiotics, and synbiotics during pregnancy or lactation on the intestinal microbiota of children born by cesarean section: a systematic review. *Nutrients.* 2022 Jan 14;14(2):341.

[181] Liu A, Chen S, et al. Probiotics improve gastrointestinal function and life quality in pregnancy. *Nutrients.* 2021 Nov 3;13(11):3931.

[182] Marzorati M, Van den Abbeele P, et al. Treatment with a spore-based probiotic containing five strains of Bacillus induced changes in the metabolic activity and community composition of the gut microbiota in a SHIME® model of the human gastrointestinal system. *Food Res Int.* 2021 Nov;149:110676.

[183] Matok I, Clark S, et al. Studying the antiemetic effect of vitamin B6 for morning sickness: pyridoxine and pyridoxal are prodrugs. *J Clin Pharmacol.* 2014 Dec;54(12):1429–33.

[184] Amzajerdi A, Keshavarz M, et al. Effect of mint aroma on nausea, vomiting and anxiety in pregnant women. *J Family Med Prim Care.* 2019 Aug 28;8(8):2597–601. doi: 10.4103/jfmpc.jfmpc_480_19. PMID: 31548939; PMCID: PMC6753788.

on the stomach, not to mention more effective than folic acid.[185]

Gut Infections

Regarding nausea from various gut infections, such as H. pylori, E. coli, C. diff, etc., you should know that while antibiotics are considered the first-line therapy, you can often use natural remedies alongside or instead of antibiotics if you catch the infections right away.

One of the first signs of a gut infection can be nausea, so if you suspect that you ate food that was spoiled or coming down with something, having some of these natural remedies at the ready can be very effective if you use them right away. The chances of viral or bacterial replication are reduced if you use herbal or vitamin therapies within minutes to hours of onset. Still, as always, if you are vomiting or sick for more than 24–48 hours, you need to seek medical attention.

Vitamin D: This has its own set of antimicrobial peptides that it makes in the body, and it is very helpful at mitigating most any type of illness, including infections. A short-term five to seven-day course of a higher dose of vitamin D is usually the best route in this case.

Oregano: This is probably my favorite herb at the first sign of belly illness, and you can use capsules or oregano oil. Because it is so strong, you should only use it for a few days in a row generally and follow label suggestions because they vary in dose.

Cardamom: A very beneficial spice because it is antimicrobial and dampens down nausea. You can make cardamom tea or buy cardamom capsules.

Caraway: This is antimicrobial and is often combined with mint to help ease stomach discomfort.

Peppermint: This also has antimicrobial properties against E. coli and is an effective anti-nausea aid.

---

[185] Houghton LA, Sherwood KL, Pawlosky R, Ito S, O'Connor DL. [6S]-5-Methyltetrahydrofolate is at least as effective as folic acid in preventing a decline in blood folate concentrations during lactation. Am J Clin Nutr. 2006 Apr;83(4):842-50.

Licorice: Helps the body fight infections and is soothing to the stomach. Just make sure to choose the DGL licorice if you plan on taking licorice for more than a couple of days.

Mullein: A great herb to help fight infections, even dampening inflammation.

Slippery elm: Helps to soothe the gut lining and provides a protective barrier in the gut against unwanted invaders.

Marshmallow root: similar to slippery elm in that it helps increase the stomach's mucus lining, which helps protect the body from infections.

Turmeric: This is not only anti-inflammatory but helps the body fight off harmful bacteria. Having some turmeric tea, adding turmeric to soups, and supplementing turmeric can be helpful for nausea.

Garlic: A potent antimicrobial herb that everyone should have in their cabinet. Using a lot of garlic helps fight unwanted infections. Just be aware that some people don't tolerate garlic due to its fermentability in the gut. Aged garlic works better in this case, and you can buy supplements of this form.

Activated charcoal: A remedy that many travelers use if they get an infectious bug to help reduce or minimize nausea or diarrhea. Learn more about it in Chapter 7.

Medication-Induced Nausea

As I mentioned, almost any prescription or over-the-counter medication can cause nausea. Even medications for heartburn can ironically cause nausea in some people, such as Pepcid. This section is to make you aware of the side effects of medications, and the main goal is to minimize your intake of any conventional drug therapies if possible. Review with your doctor or healthcare provider if your medications are absolutely necessary. Taking multiple medications simultaneously increases your risk of bad nausea side effects.

Common medications that cause nausea are:

- Antibiotics
- Pain medications
- Antidepressants
- Pepcid
- Other antacids like calcium carbonate
- Iron
- Ibuprofen
- Aspirin
- Tylenol
- Blood pressure medications like Nifedipine
- Chemotherapy

It is generally advised to take any medications with food, and supplements and remedies that may help minimize or stop nausea associated with these medications include:

Glutamine: This can help heal the gut lining so that you can tolerate medications better. Just make sure to start with a low dose. Refer to Chapter 7 for more information about how to dose glutamine.

Probiotics: Help to reduce nausea and vomiting from antibiotics and help rebuild the gut so that your medications may become more tolerable.

Cannabis: Can be given as a suppository to prevent the feelings of getting high and prevents nausea that can come along with cannabis itself. See also Chapter 7.

Ginger: Helps just about every kind of nausea, and this is no exception. It is also very safe. [186] [187]

If you are taking pain medications that cause stomach issues, you should definitely consider alternative natural pain relievers such as:

Turmeric: A natural anti-inflammatory that is clinically proven to reduce

[186] Ding M, Leach M, et al. The effectiveness and safety of ginger for pregnancy-induced nausea and vomiting: a systematic review. *Women Birth.* 2013 Mar;26(1):e26–30.

[187] Viljoen E, Visser J, et al. A systematic review and meta-analysis of the effect and safety of ginger in the treatment of pregnancy-associated nausea and vomiting. *Nutr J.* 2014 Mar 19;13:20.

many kinds of pain.

Boswellia/frankincense: Dampens inflammation and pain and works well alongside turmeric.

Ginger: Like its relative turmeric, this is also helpful for many kinds of pain, especially gut pain.

FSM therapy: I highly encourage *The Resonance Effect* by Carol McMakin to learn about how this therapy is changing how pain is being treated.

Cannabis: Can be extremely beneficial as a standalone for pain. It can be given as a suppository to prevent the feelings of getting high.

Heat and ice: Alternating heat therapies and ice packs are beneficial for almost any kind of physical pain.

Vitamin D: Vitamin D or other nutrient deficiency can cause pain, so this can be a simple fix. You MUST check your vitamin D levels at least twice a year for the best health, regardless.

N-acetylglucosamine: This is especially beneficial for dampening inflammation and pain in the gut. Read more about it in Chapter 7.

Fish oil: Also a natural anti-inflammatory, and most people need more omega-3 fats in their diets anyway.

Acupuncture: A very effective tool for pain relief for many kinds of pain, such as radiculopathy or pinched nerves.

Hypnotherapy: When pain in the body comes from our brain (it always does), clinical hypnotherapy can greatly help. I highly recommend using this for just about any health issue, but make sure to find a clinical hypnotherapist that has extensive training and excellent reviews.

Topical creams: Many natural creams are available for pain relief; see page 309 for recommendations.

Keep in mind that not all herbal therapies work for everyone. If you don't tolerate turmeric, for example, don't take it.

Case Study: Reducing Pain and Nausea the Natural Way

Tracy was about at her wit's end because she struggled with IBS and indigestion, and significant joint pain. For these conditions, she had been given prescription and over-the-counter medications a try. While the pain relievers like ibuprofen helped her joint pain, she was left with a lot of nausea and worsened symptoms of IBS and indigestion, which wasn't relieved by Pepcid® or pantoprazole. Her nausea medication (ondansetron) worked to reduce her nausea but left her feeling tired and with frequent headaches and constipation. Additionally, she was worried about taking vitamins because she was worried they would make her more nauseated.

After encouragement, Tracy agreed to take a natural B-vitamin complex along with a broad spectrum multivitamin with minerals at her dinner meal to make up for her nutrient losses due to stress, medications, and digestive issues. She was encouraged and pleasantly surprised because these vitamins didn't make her more nauseated like her previous vitamins. Because of this, she was very brave about wanting to try and eliminate her ibuprofen, nausea, and stomach acid medications so she gave the following regimen a try.

- A natural vitamin with minerals (discontinued the extra B-complex after two weeks because she was feeling better and more energetic).
- Beef liver and beef intestines supplement daily.
- Makes a gallon of ginger and cardamom or Tulsi tea to sip on throughout the week for nausea reduction and stress management.
- First thing in the morning, adds colostrum powder to a smoothie to heal the gut.
- Adds fresh sauerkraut daily to her salad or soup for probiotic benefits and to dampen stress.
- Keeps peppermint gelcaps handy for nausea symptoms.
- Takes marshmallow root capsules daily for gut soothing and healing and to increase gut mucus lining.
- Daily meditation and stress management.
- Uses charcoal instead of pantoprazole if she feels any heartburn or

indigestion symptoms break through.
- Takes a low dose cannabis tincture at bedtime to help with stress and sleep.
- Eliminates inflammatory foods like sugar and gluten.

After a week, Tracy was pleased to report that her joint pain was better, she was managing her nausea much better and was able to go without ondansetron and only needed ibuprofen once daily. After two weeks, she added turmeric for her joint pain and was able to eliminate the use of ibuprofen altogether. She was also pleased that her headaches were mostly gone and she had more energy throughout the day. She's also pleased to report that she sleeps better than ever and feels much calmer during the day.

11

Chapter 11

Constipation: Ease Your Distress

Constipation is when bowel movements pass too slowly through the colon, making them hard, dry, and/or difficult to pass. This condition isn't a disorder itself but is triggered by many health issues or lifestyle issues, as we will discuss next. For best health, it is ideal to pass a bowel movement once daily, and often constipation means only passing a couple per week.

It can happen to anyone, but some people are more prone to it, even in childhood, than others. If your constipation started as a child, it may seem normal and nearly impossible to fix, especially if you never figured out the cause. Regardless, it is important to manage this condition to improve your health overall.

Constipation is painful and annoying, but it also increases the risk of other diseases, such as colorectal cancer, Parkinson's disease, high blood pressure, asthma, allergies, heart disease, and more. Conventional medicine doesn't have any great approaches to fixing the issue either. Laxatives and stool softeners, while helpful for alleviating the issue temporarily, don't get to the real issue at hand. But knowing the root cause of your constipation can make it easier for you to figure out the best approaches to help alleviate the issue and to help prevent health issues down the road.

Advisory: When to Seek Help

If you have prolonged bouts of constipation, it can create serious issues like fecal impaction, obstruction, hemorrhoids, and more. You should seek medical help if you have vomiting, persistent abdominal pain, blood in your stool, persistent constipation, or severe bloating.

Root Causes

There are many causes of chronic constipation, and it is important to identify the main contributing factors for you. If you haven't been able to sort this out yet, here are some common possible causes. Many people often have one or more of these causes simultaneously.

Dehydration

Having too little fluid intake is a common cause of constipation and discomfort. Generally speaking, an ideal fluid intake ranges between 8–12 cups per day. However, there is a high amount of variation from person to person due to many factors, such as the types of foods you eat, the amount you perspire, your age, medications, and more. Still, most people should drink plenty of fluids, like herbal tea, water, coffee, etc., throughout the day to help prevent constipation.

Stress

Stress causes the nerves in the digestive tract to release more hormones and neurotransmitters like serotonin. This can result in diarrhea and constipation, depending on where the nerves are overactive in the gut. Managing stress and anxiety in your life is a cornerstone to relieving constipation in this case and can also be done through diet changes and supplements to help alleviate stress.

Abdominal Surgeries

Surgery can lead to **adhesions** in the gut, which makes it so that the muscles of the gut don't work properly. Abdominal massage can be helpful for some people, and others are helped by frequency-specific microcurrents. Even the Cleveland Clinic uses these techniques for many conditions such as this. Learn more here https://frequencyspecific.com/abdominal-pain-and-pelvic-adhesions-dr-carolyn-mcmakin/

SIBO

If you have an overgrowth of some types of bacteria in the gut, such as methane-producing bacteria, this makes you more prone to IBS constipation and SIBO (see also Chapter 13).

Slow Transit

Slow gut transit or slow muscle movements are due to issues in the enteric nervous system. Relaxation techniques are helpful, including yoga, hypnotherapy, herbal therapies outlined in Chapter 7, breathing exercises, singing, laughing, socializing, etc.

Redundant Colon

This a condition that some people are born with, and it essentially is an extra-long colon that bends or kinks in the wrong places because of it. This can result in serious constipation throughout one's life. The extra length of the colon may cause slowing of bowel movements because it delays the migratory motor complex in the gut. Intermittent fasting may help this condition. Artichoke leaf extract and ginger may be helpful for people who have this too.

Medications

Common medications such as antibiotics, prescription pain medications, antihistamines, dietary supplements like iron and calcium, antidepressants, and even fiber supplements, if done improperly without plenty of fluids and gentle introduction, can cause constipation.

Imbalanced Diet (for you)

There is no single right diet for constipation because people are genetically different. If you notice certain foods cause constipation for you, please avoid them. This can ironically be so-called healthy foods like whole wheat, vegetables, other grains, and dairy products.

Imbalanced Microbiome

A lack of healthy bacteria in the gut can cause or contribute to bacteria symptoms. This is where probiotics and prebiotics can come in really helpful.

Food Sensitivities and Allergies

As discussed previously, food sensitivities and allergies are quite common and can cause constipation. Following an elimination diet is very doable-you can do it for a few weeks to help determine your main sensitivities.

Lack of Exercise

Have you ever been sitting on an airplane or in a car for hours and noticed you are constipated after you do this? This is because the lack of exercise during travel causes intestinal movements to drastically be reduced. Generally speaking, exercise helps stimulate normal bowel movements and shouldn't be neglected.

Autoimmune/Nerve Conditions

Any condition that damages the nerves or impairment of the nerves, such as diabetes, multiple sclerosis, Parkinson's disease, enteric nervous system disorders, spinal cord damage, etc. The main goal in helping these conditions is eating foods that support nerve health and can include an autoimmune diet like *The Wahls Protocol* Dr. Terry Wahls.

Diet Strategies for Constipation

Believe me when I say there is no one-size-fits-all for diets that can reduce constipation. For example, fiber can help some people, while it can compound the problem in others. Finding the right diet for you may take trial and error, but it is worth it. But you must keep an open mind about what is good for you and what is not. This means you will likely need to filter everything you've heard in the news about "healthy" foods.

For example, some people who have struggled with constipation for years on a fiber-rich diet find that switching to a **ketogenic diet** alleviated their constipation concerns.

Did You Know . . . Beware of Associations in Studies

Remember, studies that call fiber healthy for the gut are usually based on associations. You can make associations with anything, such as this: gray cars are more likely to stall on the side of the road. While this is silly, statistics make it easy to make false associations like this. False associations with food and disease risk happen all the time due to bias in the people reporting their diet history, incidental luck, and the scientists reporting the statistics. If a food causes bloating, you should probably minimize or avoid it if you have constipation.

Foods that cause bloat are usually fermentable fibers like beans, wheat, other grains, fruits, vegetables, onion, and garlic. Even avocados are sadly high in fermentable fibers. Dairy products can contain fermentable fibers, too, especially milk and ice cream, but less so with cheese and yogurt. These fermentable fibers are called FODMAPS. Many popular websites and research are dedicated to helping people minimize these fermentable foods. The very popular book *The Microbiome Connection* by Dr. Pimentel is also dedicated to this.

Bloating isn't benign if you have constipation. The extra air in the gut causes the intestinal muscles to be ineffective in moving waste out of the body for some people. In essence, bloating due to some fibers can make constipation worse.

That said, the foods that tend to cause the least GI distress for people with constipation are typically organically raised and pasture-fed meats like 100 percent grass-finished meats, pastured chicken, wild-caught fish, unprocessed fats, and oils like extra-virgin olive oil. In fact, extra virgin olive oil itself can help alleviate constipation, and I recommend having at least 3 tablespoons a day to help lubricate the gut. It is rich in polyphenols that help fuel healthy bacteria in the colon too. To complicate things, onions may cause bloating when raw, but when slow-cooked and blended into a pureed soup may be perfectly tolerated.

Building your diet from foods you tolerate can be a good starting place. For me, having plain whole milk yogurt, bananas, green leafy vegetables with olive oil and vinegar, slow-cooked chicken or beef (bone-in), bone-broth soups, fish, sushi, rice, carrots, lots of mushrooms, sweet potatoes, herbs, spices, and stews are some of the best foods I can eat. Avoiding gluten, beans, and unfermented milk as much as possible keeps my gut happy. But again, a lot depends on your genetics, and what works for me won't necessarily work for you.

Whatever you decide, stick with it for at least three weeks and keep food records to help you determine the best course. Systematically add back suspected trigger foods one at a time and be patient. Add only one food back at a time over three days to better understand how this food affects you. Additionally, consider using some of the following herbs, nutrients, and other supplements if you have constipation to help you get at the root of your constipation issues.

Natural Supplements for Constipation Pain

Constipation can be painful, annoying, and downright distracting from your daily life. When looking for natural remedies to alleviate pain and discomfort, there are a few to keep on hand that may be a godsend.

The following three supplements don't really fit into the herb category but are all-natural ways to potentially help you feel better.

NAG

NAG, or n-acetylglucosamine, can help reduce abdominal pain due to inflammatory bowel diseases in 60 percent of those suffering from this condition. This natural supplement helps to increase the thickness of the mucin lining in the gut, which is the protective barrier. This supplement can also reduce harmful bacterial biofilms, which may help alleviate many kinds of digestive issues.

Research shows that doses of up to 6g of NAG daily are safe and effective.[188] A more common dose for NAG is around 700 mg. Remember that NAG is made from shellfish, so if you are allergic to shellfish, avoid it.

Glutamine

Glutamine is a natural amino acid that fuels intestinal cells, improves the gut microbiome, and helps heal the gut lining. Doing so can even help alleviate constipation symptoms in some people. Many people feel like it helps rather quickly and even reduces sugar cravings. It's a huge help for bloating, which can be a big problem in people with constipation.

---

[188] Ali R, Irfan M, et al. Efficacy of natural formulation containing activated charcoal, calcium sennosides, peppermint oil, fennel oil, rhubarb extract, and purified sulfur (Nucarb®) in relieving constipation. *Cureus.* 2021 Oct 1;13(10):e18419.

Having glutamine around the home is a smart idea because it can help with so many digestive issues. Using it periodically during times of digestive distress can be very helpful. For example, using it over three to five days is typically all you need.

Glutamine tends to work best on an empty stomach, but this can be nauseating for some people, so you could sip on it after eating a small amount of food. I recommend glutamine powder so you can sip slowly for about an hour. A good starting point is around 5 g per day.

Collagen

Unlike laxatives that blast the gut, supplements like collagen may have a subtler and nourishing effect that can help result in more normal bowel movements when used over time. This is because collagen helps heal the gut lining, helps improve the microbiome, and even helps to increase the fuel for your gut cells, called butyrate. Additionally, it helps the liver make bile to improve digestive processes. Additionally, collagen draws water towards it, so it may help soften bowel movements too.

A side benefit of collagen is that it can improve skin health and even can help reduce cholesterol levels, according to some studies. Choose a collagen supplement from healthy animals, such as 100 percent grass-fed beef and wild-caught fish.

Activated Charcoal

Usually used as a rescue treatment for all sorts of belly issues, activated charcoal is a natural supplement that can reduce constipation pain in some people because it absorbs gas in the gut. One study found that activated charcoal as part of an herbal supplement called Nucarb reduced the severity of constipation by as much as 81 percent.[189] This supplement is unavailable for most people now, but it contains activated charcoal, senna, peppermint oil, fennel oil, rhubarb extract, and purified sulfur. It is impossible to know which ingredients provide the most relief or if they work together synergistically.

But starting slowly as activated charcoal at high doses can be constipating in a small number of people. I suggest starting with 1 capsule, adding 1 dose of senna and peppermint, and testing how it makes you feel.

Chlorella

A type of algae, chlorella, is an extremely helpful supplement that can reduce constipation for many people. But it doesn't work for everyone. And not everyone feels wonderful when they first try it. This is because it is so cleansing that it can create a healing reaction in the body. Some people feel better after about a week, but it is usually a little worse before feeling better.

Hence it helps to start small. Typically, the package directions will say to take 6 tablets a day or a tablespoon a day. Starting with a third of that dose is my recommendation, and work your way up over several days to get to the package suggested dose.

It is well worth your time because many people report having more energy and looking younger, too, and chlorella nourishes the body. Do note, though, chlorella is considered a seafood, so there is a remote chance that if you have a seafood allergy, you could react to algae. Also, find broken cell wall chlorella, which most are.

---

[189] Bundy R, Walker A, et al. Artichoke leaf extract reduces symptoms of irritable bowel syndrome and improves quality of life in otherwise healthy volunteers suffering from concomitant dyspepsia: A subset analysis. *J Altern Complement Med.* 2004 Aug;10(4):667–9.

Herbs that Help Constipation

If you have constipation, herbal therapies are great because they can work on multiple root causes of this condition. Most of these herbs are multi-taskers: they help dampen inflammation, reduce stress and anxiety, and can help heal the gut and microbiome all at once. In other words, they are usually gentle and effective options for almost everyone.

Triphala: The Multipurpose Herbal Blend

Triphala is an Ayurvedic multipurpose herbal remedy for constipation and works to lubricate, cleanse, reduce inflammation, and provide bulk to the stool simultaneously. Because it is a blend of three herbs, it works on many aspects of digestive health.

Using Triphala can take a week or two to work, but many people say this herbal blend works for constipation when nothing else ever would. Some people even say it helps severe constipation, which comes with issues like spinal cord injury-induced constipation.

Doses of the herbal blend usually range between 600–1000 mg per day. You can find Triphala on Fullscript and at reputable herbal dispensaries such as health food stores.

Bitters that Promote Digestive Function

Many herbs are considered bitters and are traditionally used to help prevent and treat constipation symptoms. They are known to help increase digestive enzyme flow from the gallbladder, so they support regular bowel movements too.

Herbs like gentian root, dandelion root, barberry, and artichoke are considered bitters. Additionally, fennel seeds, burdock root, turmeric root, cardamom, dill, caraway, and cardamom are often added to bitters supplements to support the speed of the digestive tract. Most bitters supplements have a combination of these herbs. It is best to take bitters before you eat to help improve the digestive process during your mealtime.

Herbs That Stimulate Intestinal Muscles

If you have had sluggish bowels your whole life, odds are, your intestinal muscles may move too slowly. Some lifestyle tips to help this include intermittent fasting. Intermittent fasting helps to coordinate the **migratory motor complex** of the gut, thereby helping to reduce constipation. Additionally, some herbs help increase the muscle movements of the gut too. They are:

- Ginger
- Senna
- Caraway
- Aloe

Like many herbs, these have multiple benefits on the gut, like reducing inflammation, healing the gut, and stimulating muscle movements. Refer to Chapter 7 for more details about how to use these herbs. Other herbs like cardamom, turmeric, and ginger improve circulation and bolster immunity, which may indirectly help with bowel movements too. Contrary to popular opinion, herbs that stimulate the intestines are not habit-forming. And when senna is combined with fiber therapy, it works better than strong laxative medications like lactulose.

Herbs That Balance and Calm

As I described before, stress can do a number on the gut and can contribute to constipation for many people. So, herbs are a logical choice to help balance out the negative effects of stress hormones and the bowel movement issues that go along with them.

Cannabis: A variant that contains the full spectrum of both THC and CBD can be very calming if used appropriately. Many people find that cannabis helps ease their gut issues, including constipation. But go low and take it slow, as reviewed in Chapter 7.

Fennel seeds: These are an all-around rock star for gut health and are calming and balancing for the gut.

Iberogast: A blend of herbs that can be calming and relaxing to the gut, making bowel movements easier to pass.

Mullein: Often underused, this is such a beneficial herb and is traditionally used as a treatment for constipation.

Red raspberry leaf: This has balancing effects on hormones and as a healthy gut tonic. It is a safe and popular tea (although it should be avoided until late in the third trimester of pregnancy) that you can use daily.

Slippery elm/marshmallow root: These are both very soothing and calming herbs that help heal the gut lining, so they help most anyone balance out stress.

Tulsi: A great-all around herb that is safe for daily use. It helps calm the mind and the gut.

Milk thistle: Promotes bowel regularity and is rich in antioxidants that dampen inflammation in the gut as well.

Herbs That Reduce Gas

Some herbs can help reduce gas production in the gut, so manage multiple symptoms of this condition. While many herbs have this function, the most well-known herbs to help reduce gas include fennel seeds, bay leaves, caraway, cardamom, chamomile, coriander, dill, ginger, milk thistle, peppermint, and turmeric. In many cultures, it is common to use these remedies, and you can chew up several fennel or caraway seeds for a quick fix or make tea out of any of these herbs and spices. They are all very safe to try but read more information in Chapter 7 if you want to know more about how to use each of these herbs.

Alternatively, use Iberogast as a supplement for constipation. It contains many herbs and is clinically verified for its gut health benefits. Or, you can find most of these herbs in supplement forms these days as well, but make sure to follow package directions and use them only as needed because while effective, you could, in theory, overdo them if you take them all of the time.

Another clinically proven supplement for gas-related constipation is called MegaGuard (page 307), which is a combination of standardized artichoke leaf, GutGuard licorice, and standardized ginger at 20 percent.[190] [191]

Magnesium for Prevention

When it comes to constipation, magnesium works exceptionally well. It gets to the root cause of many forms of constipation! Magnesium helps to prevent constipation, increases fluid in the gut, binds unwanted compounds like oxalates, relaxes the gut muscles so that they can move more effectively, and helps to heal a leaky gut. In addition, magnesium supports a healthy bacteria content for the microbiome.

A couple of other reminders: If you don't eat leafy greens, nuts, and seeds daily, you run a very high risk of magnesium deficiency. Many medications may also rob you of magnesium. And blood tests of magnesium levels are notoriously inaccurate unless you specifically ask your doctor to measure red blood cell magnesium levels. Given that most Americans are low in magnesium intake anyway, magnesium supplements are a logical choice for constipation.

Regarding constipation, a couple of forms of magnesium work the best: magnesium oxide and magnesium citrate. Magnesium citrate has a milder laxative effect than magnesium oxide, so depending on your situation, you may want to choose one form over the other. Magnesium citrate also is absorbed better, so it may be the best choice if you are also suspecting you are low in magnesium or suffer from muscle cramps or poor sleep.

Other forms of magnesium serve better as nutritional magnesium, such as

[190] Kwon Y, Son D, et al. A review of the pharmacological efficacy and safety of licorice root from corroborative clinical trial findings. *J Med Food.* 2020 Jan;23(1):12–20.

[191] Holtmann G, Adam B, et al. Efficacy of artichoke leaf extract in the treatment of patients with functional dyspepsia: A six-week placebo-controlled, double-blind, multicentre trial. *Aliment Pharmacol Ther.* 2003 Dec;18(11-12):1099–105.

magnesium glycinate and magnesium malate. Because of this, they are less likely to help with constipation, however. Also, a powder or capsule form will be more effective than a tablet form of magnesium. But as a general rule of thumb, you should start with a low dose, such as 300 mg of magnesium citrate or magnesium oxide, per day to see if that amount helps. If not, increase the dose, but if you take more than 500 mg per day, make sure to get your red blood cell magnesium levels checked.

You can find a high-quality magnesium supplement with magnesium citrate, magnesium oxide, and magnesium malate on Fullscript or at local herbal dispensaries.

Probiotics and Prebiotics

As you now know, probiotics are dynamic multi-taskers when it comes to bowel habits, meaning they help many aspects of gut function to result in a net result of fewer constipation symptoms overall. But, they can vary in their effectiveness depending on the root cause of your constipation. For example, if you have SIBO-related constipation, some probiotics may make you feel worse, such as some strains of Bifidobacterium.

Overall, the research consensus is that most strains of probiotics are helpful with most kinds of constipation.[192] My favorite strains are Bacillus strains, as reviewed in Chapter 8. This is primarily because they are often the best tolerated and don't take nearly as high of concentrations to have a beneficial effect. But, again, you may want to try a variety of strains because everyone's microbiome is different. Just make sure to give it some time—a couple of weeks or so, and you should know if it will be helpful for you or not. More types of strains and higher concentrations are generally better too. For moderate to severe constipation, probiotic therapy isn't usually enough, but it is a good add-on therapy to improve overall gut health.

---

[192] Dimidi E, Christodoulides S, et al. The effect of probiotics on functional constipation in adults: A systematic review and meta-analysis of randomized controlled trials. *Am J Clin Nutr.* 2014 Oct;100(4):1075--84.

Probiotics help to heal a leaky gut, so by fixing your constipation with healthy probiotics and a healthy diet, you are also helping your whole body and mind feel better. However, sometimes starting a probiotic can result in some temporary gas, bloating, and, ironically, constipation. If this happens, try to stay the course, but if you need to cut back on the dose, you can break open a capsule and take a ¼ capsule, and then gradually increase your dose. Or you can try a very gentle probiotic; see page 307 for recommendations.

But, when it comes to *prebiotics*, they can be helpful but also pesky to try, as reviewed in Chapter 8. I suggest starting with a very low dose, such as 1 g per day, from whole-food sources such as medicinal mushrooms and beetroot extract. Or pectin is a pretty gentle type of prebiotic to try. You certainly can try some chicory fiber, but start very slowly, or you may end up gassier and more bloated than you were in the first place. In other words, it's best to try prebiotics once your bowel movements are in a more normal pattern. They can add to the bulk of stools, but this isn't always a good thing if you are backed up.

Digestive Enzymes

Another great multi-tasker supplement for gut health, including constipation, is digestive enzymes. They can help with constipation because they help make nutrients more digestible and less gas-producing. There aren't ten studies showing that digestive enzymes help, but they help with the awful symptoms of constipation, like gas, bloating, and pain.

Other Helpful Supplements for Managing Constipation

Last but not least, several other supplements can help manage the root causes of constipation. They include quercetin, vitamin C, MCT oil, and multivitamins with minerals.

Quercetin: Promotes gut healing and bowel regularity and dampens down inflammation.

Vitamin C: Helps immune function, and similar to magnesium, it pulls water towards it, making bowel movements pass more easily. For constipation, typically use greater than 1 g of vitamin C.

MCT Oil: Reduces candida growth, helps reduce the growth of harmful bacteria, and stimulates the muscle movements of the gut. It is a quick fix for constipation, but you may want to be close to a bathroom if you are new to using this supplement. Drink it slowly, starting with a teaspoon—do not chug it. Even better yet, add it to your coffee or tea and sip it slowly.

MCT oil should be in the caprylic acid form because if it contains lauric acid, it may negatively affect some people's cholesterol levels.

Multivitamins and minerals: These help constipation indirectly because a lack of almost any nutrient can make the microbiome out of balance. You may also need to add vitamin D and K2 to get optimal amounts of those nutrients.

Case Study: Constipation Relief Comes Naturally

Sarah struggled with acid reflux and redundant colon because she was born with a kink in her large intestine. This kink caused many digestive problems, including significant gut pain and constipation, followed by occasional bouts of diarrhea. It also seemed to be part of the cause of her frequent acid reflux. Her doctor told her that the kink impaired her gut muscle movements and recommended using laxatives. Unfortunately, over-the-counter laxatives caused her much more belly pain than not taking them, so she suffered in silence with constipation and pain for years.

Interested in herbal and nutritional therapies, Sarah decided to eat a healing diet along with taking n-acetylglucosamine for her pain which helped to reduce the frequency of gut pain significantly. She also decided to use digestive enzymes to reduce her acid reflux symptoms when she was eating meals and she also added in Iberogast® herbal supplement as needed for heartburn. This combination worked well and didn't cause any side effects for her acid reflux while also reducing constipation symptoms. Sarah also added senna tea which was much gentler on her system than over-the-counter laxatives, so it further reduced the constipation and the diarrhea symptoms that followed using previous strategies for her constipation.

12

Chapter 12

Diarrhea: Simple Strategies That Work

It seems like having healthy regular bowel movements is becoming rarer as gut issues become increasingly common. In fact, most people have multiple bouts of diarrhea per year, and some have it more or less all of the time. In this chapter, you'll learn about different types, what causes it, and how to improve your diet and replenish your system with nutrients and supplements to overcome it. By doing so, you can often tackle the root causes of diarrhea and feel better soon.

Diarrhea Defined

If you have diarrhea, you have three or more loose or watery stools per day. Many people have loose stools daily but don't have this frequency of loose stools: so that is not technically considered diarrhea. However, loose stools, in general, can still be a sign of imbalances in the body, so it is important to figure out how to resolve this issue.

There are three main types of diarrhea: fatty, watery, and inflammatory.

Fatty diarrhea: If you have fatty diarrhea, you will often know it because it is foul smelling and will have small amounts of fat that float at the top of the water in the toilet. The causes of fatty diarrhea are many, including gut surgery, parasites, pancreatic insufficiency, circulation issues to the gut (ischemia), and low bile levels.

Watery diarrhea: This is caused by excess carbohydrate intake or carbohydrate intolerances (i.e., fructose or sucrose), alcohol, increased gut muscle movements, infections, food sensitivities and intolerances, bile acid malabsorption, anxiety, and IBS.

Inflammatory diarrhea. This relates to inflammatory diseases like Crohn's, ulcerative colitis, diverticulosis, infections, food sensitivities, certain kinds of cancer, and radiation treatment.

However, some conditions, like celiac disease or Crohn's disease, can have all three types of diarrhea at once. Talk about a difficult experience. Luckily, there are many natural ways to reduce diarrhea by improving your diet, bolstering your immune system, calming the mind, and decreasing inflammation through diet and supplements.

Advisory: When to Seek Help

While this chapter is meant to help you prevent diarrhea and loose stool symptoms or minimize them, there are times when you need to seek medical attention. If you have diarrhea for more than two days or also have a fever, severe pain, mental status changes, dark urine, or blood in your bowel movements, you should consult with your healthcare provider right away.

Diet Strategies to Reduce Diarrhea Symptoms

Diarrhea is perhaps easier to fix with diet than constipation in some situations because you can add bulk to help and healing compounds to calm the gut down. By getting your diet and lifestyle into shape, you can help minimize or eliminate these symptoms by combining them with the right supplements. However, if you have a rare condition called **short gut syndrome**, these tips don't necessarily all apply to you.

Avoid alcohol, sugars, and refined carbohydrates: These obvious diarrhea culprits cause watery diarrhea and should be eliminated or avoided as much as possible. This includes all sweet treats, sweet beverages, and most bread, crackers, pastries, etc.

Eat healing foods: There is a reason that your grandmother fed you nourishing chicken vegetable soup when you were sick. If made well with bone broth, it provides healing collagen, electrolytes, and nutrients that help you recover from diarrhea. Slow-cooked meats with root vegetables like sweet potatoes and greens are your best bets.

Replenish lost nutrients and digestive factors: This is a step that most people sadly skip, but if you have had diarrhea, the odds are that you are low in vitamins, minerals, digestive enzymes, and more. You will heal from diarrhea symptoms much more quickly if you have the proper nutrients to support your immune system and heal your gut. We will dive into more of this topic later in this chapter.

Identify and eliminate food sensitivities and intolerances: Common food sensitivities can cause diarrhea and include gluten, dairy, corn, soy, eggs, nuts, and shellfish. By following an elimination diet or a modified elimination diet, you can use my *Elimination Diet Journal* for this or *The Elimination Diet* by Tom Malterre.

Try adding bulk: Prebiotics and soluble fibers can be a big help by helping make your stools more formed. The only case where you will want to avoid more bulk is if you have low bile levels, as you will learn about next.

Determine if you are low or high in bile: It is important to identify if you have low or high bile, and it's fairly easy to tell if you suffer from diarrhea. Low bile levels result in pasty, pale-colored stools. High bile, or bile malabsorption, results in very smelly poops; fatty foods usually trigger diarrhea and bloating symptoms with bile malabsorption. With high bile levels, you will probably need to ensure you don't have gallstones. But there are some natural remedies to prevent or manage these, too, as long as you aren't having severe gallbladder issues (Chapter 16).

Himalayan pink salt: If you have ongoing diarrhea, you shouldn't limit salt because sodium is an electrolyte depleted by diarrhea unless advised by your healthcare practitioner. Too little salt can impair your gut muscles.

Whole Food Supplements for Diarrhea Symptoms

In this section, you will learn how to use various whole-food supplements for diarrhea symptoms. These supplements are very safe and life-changing when used consistently, using the right doses, and at the right times.

The best part about your gut cells and healing is that the average lifespan of gut cells is only five days. By nourishing your gut cells, you can dramatically impact diarrhea symptoms fairly quickly if you have already followed the diet steps described above.

But, your baseline diet impacts which supplements will help the most. So, for example, if you never eat fish, you could be low in omega-3 fats that are critical for intestinal cell function, and supplementing will be helpful long term. If you regularly eat fish, this may not be the first priority for adding it as a supplement. And if you eat bone-in meats with bone broth, you may not benefit from a collagen supplement as much as other remedies discussed in this chapter.

A basic healing combination that I recommend for most people is bovine colostrum, organ meats, glutamine, digestive enzymes, probiotics, vitamin D3 with vitamin K2, omega-3 fats, and a natural multivitamin with minerals. But, you should read through them all in Chapter 6 and decide what is best for you based on your health needs and special diet and gut concerns.

Keep in mind that you don't necessarily have to stay on this regimen forever; only during the healing process. But, you may find ones like bovine colostrum, organ meats, and multivitamin with minerals are indispensable as a daily routine for preventing diarrhea and overall gut health.

Bovine Colostrum

Bovine colostrum is one of my favorite dual-purpose supplements and one I won't live without. Research shows that it is effective in helping treat acute diarrhea and for preventing diarrhea in multiple clinical studies, which is no surprise given how immune-boosting it is.[193] [194]It also helps get to the root cause of inflammatory bowel disease conditions through its rich lactoferrin content, growth factors, immune cells, lysozyme, and immunoglobulin. More than that, it contains ninety known healing compounds, which gobble up infectious bacteria and viruses and even bolster your own innate immunity. Also, research shows it helps heal a leaky gut, which is common in people who suffer from diarrhea.[195]

You only need to avoid bovine colostrum if you have a milk allergy. It is fine for people who are lactose intolerant because it only contains a trace.

To use bovine colostrum, it is best to start with 1 teaspoon a day and increase it as tolerated to 1 tablespoon per day. You can mix it in water or put it in any cold beverage. But avoid adding it to hot beverages because it can deactivate the immune compounds. Using it as a powder is best because, as you may recall, your gut begins in your mouth, and the healing compounds start here. If you absolutely can't handle the idea of using it in powder form, capsules are available (see page 305 for recommendations).

Collagen

In Chapter 3, I reviewed the extensive benefits of collagen for gut health. If you have diarrhea symptoms, collagen can help eliminate several root causes, such as inflammation and lack of gut-healing amino acids. It is healing, anti-inflammatory, helps the body make bile, and dampens inflammation. Collagen is one of the reasons that Grandma's homemade chicken soup is so healthy as a diarrhea remedy.

---

[193] Barakat S, Meheissen M, et al. Bovine colostrum in the treatment of acute diarrhea in children: A double-blinded randomized controlled trial. *J Trop Pediatr.* 2020 Feb 1;66(1):46–55.

[194] Huppertz H, Rutkowski S, et al. Bovine colostrum ameliorates diarrhea in infection with diarrheagenic Escherichia coli, shiga toxin-producing E. coli, and E. coli expressing intimin and hemolysin. *J Pediatr Gastroenterol Nutr.* 1999 Oct;29(4):452–6.

[195] Dziewiecka H, Buttar H, et al. A systematic review of the influence of bovine colostrum supplementation on leaky gut syndrome in athletes: Diagnostic biomarkers and future directions. *Nutrients.* 2022 Jun 17;14(12):2512.

If you don't eat collagen-rich foods daily, such as bone broth, slow-cooked bone-in meats, chicken skin, fish skin, sardines, bone broth, etc., you should consider adding a collagen or bone broth supplement. I recommend sipping collagen protein at least once daily or adding it to your soups or main dishes.

Glutamine

Glutamine is another healing compound. It is your gut wall's primary fuel source, and in times of illness or stress, the body needs a lot of glutamine. In children with diarrhea, using glutamine shortened acute diarrhea symptoms by a day, according to research.[196] Impressively, it also dramatically helps reduce IBS symptoms. It is also very helpful for healing a leaky gut and may even reduce SIBO symptoms by reducing harmful bacteria growth.

Start with 1 teaspoon of glutamine powder daily and mix it into water or any cold beverage. I recommend slowly sipping on glutamine on an empty stomach for optimal benefits. Don't gulp it because it is pretty strong, and it has more benefits if you bathe your intestinal cells throughout the day.

Organ Meats

Lacking nutrients and enzymes can cause diarrhea. For example, a lack of vitamin A, zinc, thiamine, and niacin can cause or contribute to diarrhea symptoms. Luckily, nature provides all of these when it comes to organ meats. The best organ meat for filling the gaps in nutrients is 100 percent grass-fed beef liver.

When it comes to organ meats rich in enzymes, the pancreas, intestines, and gallbladder are your best bets to support digestive function in this way, especially if you have diarrhea. Adding these three organ meat supplements is a natural game-changer for many people struggling with digestive issues

---

[196] Yalçin S, Yurdakök K, et al. Effect of glutamine supplementation on diarrhea, interleukin-8 and secretory immunoglobulin A in children with acute diarrhea. *J Pediatr Gastroenterol Nutr.* 2004 May;38(5):494–501.

and even diabetes.

Typically, you can use the dose recommended on the label for grass-fed beef liver. Still, with the other organ meats like the pancreas, intestines, and gallbladder, I suggest starting with half the recommended dose and taking them with meals. You can increase your dose to the package recommendations after a week.

Digestive Enzymes

If you can't stomach the idea of adding in organ meats like gallbladder and pancreas to get extra enzymes in your diet, adding in digestive enzymes supplements is another great option. I reviewed a lot of the details of why digestive enzymes help the body in Chapter 7, so you can take a glance back there to review all of their beneficial effects. I've had clients that have struggled with horrible diarrhea due to gut surgeries for years and became horribly malnourished, only to find tremendous relief and regain their health when taking digestive enzymes combined with bile acids, which we will discuss next.

To add digestive enzymes for diarrhea, take broad-spectrum digestive enzyme supplements with each meal. That way, your body can break the foods down more effectively, and this helps to regulate bowel movements. Even if you forget to take the digestive enzymes until after your meal, go ahead and take it. Many meals will digest over several hours, so you may still get some relief this way.

Bile Acid

If you have diarrhea symptoms but also have pale-colored stools, the odds are that you are also low in bile. This can happen due to gallbladder surgery, and long-term diarrhea symptoms can cause it too. This is because, with diarrhea, the body fails to reabsorb bile as it should. Sadly, this lack of bile will only make your diarrhea worse because you will not absorb the foods in your diet, particularly fats and vitamins, properly. The result can be many physical symptoms over and above diarrhea, including dry skin, eczema, mood swings, and hormonal issues, to name a few.

The best bet for adding bile is gallbladder supplements or ox bile supplements. Research also shows that using a bile supplement called TUDCA is very helpful. [197] Ox bile dosage is typically 125–500 mg per meal.

On the opposite end of the spectrum, some diarrhea can be due to bile acid malabsorption. In this case, the stool color is more yellow in color. It typically hits you suddenly with diarrhea and often at nighttime. It is particularly foul-smelling. I am telling you the symptoms because it almost always is overlooked by healthcare providers. Most often, this type of diarrhea is brought on by inflammatory bowel diseases, SIBO, and celiac disease. Addressing the diet by reducing inflammatory carbohydrates, processed fats, and more, as reviewed above, is a cornerstone of treating this type of bile issue. Additionally, adding a fiber supplement is helpful, as we will discuss soon.

Medicinal Mushrooms

There is no doubt that medicinal mushrooms have hit prime time due to their powerful effects on the body. The types of mushrooms that may help digestive function range from Reishi, Chaga, Shiitake, Turkey Tail, Lion's Mane, and more.

While there are no specific guidelines for use if you have diarrhea, they are all rich in prebiotic fibers and immune-enhancing compounds, which may help control it. They are natural mood-boosters, so they may reduce stress-related diarrhea symptoms too.

However, some people don't tolerate mushrooms due to sensitivities or some of the compounds found in them. So, if you do decide to supplement

---

[197] Croce E, Golia M, et al. Razionale all'utilizzo dei sali biliari nel paziente colecistectomizzato: risultati di uno studio clinico controllato con l'impiego dell'acido tauroursodesossico lico (TUDCA) [Rationale for the use of bile salts after cholecystectomy: Results of a controlled clinical study using tauroursodeoxycholic acid (TUDCA)]. *Ann Ital Chir.* 1993 Sep-Oct;64(5):533–7. Italian.

medicinal mushrooms, go easy at first and see how your body responds. Experts in the field of medicinal mushrooms recommend mixing the mushrooms in lemon juice for 20 minutes first before eating them to make the fibers more digestible.

Personally, I find that medicinal mushrooms are definitely calming, but I don't notice a change in my bowel movements, and I use them regularly. I only include them here to let you know the options, and we all are different in terms of what our bodies respond to.

Omega-3 Fatty Acids

When adding omega-3 fatty acids, they are so helpful for almost everything, but you should know it isn't a quick fix for anything. After taking omega-3 fats, you may notice subtle but real benefits in gut symptoms like diarrhea after around six weeks. Most people are so chronically deficient that it takes this long to replenish their stores. As reviewed in Chapter 7, your best options are cod liver oil because they absorb better and contain natural vitamin A, which is particularly healing for the gut.

Probiotics and Prebiotics for Diarrhea Relief

Probiotics

Probiotics not only help alleviate constipation, but they are also great for both preventing and managing diarrhea symptoms. Because they regulate so much of how our bodies work, it is no surprise that they can reduce diarrhea symptoms too. Countless studies show that most kinds of probiotic strains work well for reducing diarrhea symptoms.

They reduce the following kinds of diarrhea:

- Stress-related diarrhea
- Antibiotic-related diarrhea
- Infectious diarrhea

I suggest trying *Bacillus* strains first because they are the gentlest to tolerate for many and don't require such high doses. But you usually can't go too far wrong, so review the various kinds of probiotics in Chapter 8. However, sometimes starting a probiotic can result in temporary gas, bloating, and, ironically, diarrhea. If this happens, try to stay the course, but if you need to cut back on the dose, you can break open a capsule and take a ¼ capsule until you can gradually increase your dose. Or you can try a very gentle probiotic; see page 307 for recommendations.

Prebiotic Fibers

One of the most effective places for prebiotic fibers in terms of gut issues is for helping treat diarrhea. The lines blur between prebiotics and fiber because they are often, but not always, one and the same. However, if you have diarrhea, you should avoid the types of fibers called insoluble fibers, which are typically the kinds found in whole grains, i.e., wheat bran, whole wheat, whole grain corn, and brown rice. You may do okay with gluten-free oats, however.

Additionally, I recommend avoiding legumes if you have diarrhea because they are a common gut irritant. I can't recommend flax seeds either unless you carefully ferment them. The best types of prebiotic fibers for diarrhea are acacia fiber, beetroot fiber, apple pectin, guar gum, and psyllium. Medicinal mushrooms, as reviewed above, also have prebiotic fibers called beta-glucan.

It is best to go with low amounts of prebiotic fibers first and remember that some people don't tolerate some kinds of prebiotic fibers, such as people with SIBO. If you have SIBO and want to try fiber, your best bet is guar gum.

I recommend starting with 1 teaspoon of prebiotic fiber daily, or between 2–4 g daily, and seeing how you do. You can increase this if you tolerate it over two days. Also, they work better when combined with probiotics.

Herbs for Diarrhea Symptoms

While herbs are often relegated, they shouldn't be. Most herbs listed below are safe and can be used daily, except for activated charcoal. The beauty is that they don't negatively interact together either, especially when used in tea forms.

Here are the most commonly used herbs to help soothe an irritated gut related to diarrhea.

Activated Charcoal: Helps bind toxins and unwanted bacteria as well as gas. For this reason, it is a great remedy, and many people use it to prevent or treat traveler's diarrhea or other infectious diarrhea. It's actually used around the world for this purpose.

Chamomile: Another great herb for reducing stress, so it dampens diarrhea symptoms for many people because of this. Having chamomile tea daily or supplements is a wonderful routine for this reason.

Cannabis: This is not just for pain, although it does help provide tremendous pain relief. It may help reduce diarrhea by relaxing gut smooth muscles, elevating the mood, reducing gut fluid secretions, and reducing inflammation and muscle spasms in the gut. Low and slow is the rule here, however.

Catnip: One of the root causes of diarrhea is stress, and because catnip is stress-busting, it may help reduce diarrhea symptoms and has been traditionally used for this purpose. Surprisingly, it makes a great tea. Serve up some for you and your cat.

Ginger: Helps alleviate both diarrhea and constipation, and that is part of why it is one of the most indispensable herbs to have around for gut health. Supplements or tea are very helpful.

Fennel: This is another multi-purpose herb. Fennel helps to regulate the bowels. Specifically, fennel helps reduce infectious types of diarrhea.

Lemon balm: Nature has many plants that serve similar functions, and similar to chamomile, lemon balm helps dampen stress and even has antimicrobial properties. It's very safe and grows like a weed, so it's nice to have some of this in your garden.

Marshmallow root/slippery elm: Both herbs are soothing to an irritated gut and help defend the body from unwanted bacteria by enhancing the mucin layer in the gut.

Red raspberry leaf: A balancing herb for gut and bowel regularity, and it even helps improve hormonal balance.

Tulsi: This is my favorite tea, and it is also good as a supplement. Because of its relaxing qualities and nutritional benefits, it may help prevent and treat diarrhea symptoms.

Vitamins and Minerals for Healthy Bowel Movements

If you have too little of just about any nutrient, it causes a disruption to gut health and can even cause diarrhea. For this reason, it makes sense to take a broad-spectrum multivitamin with minerals. Not only do these nutrients bolster your immune system to help fight off infectious diarrhea, but they also help heal the gut lining and protect the gut from oxidative damage. I recommend high-quality brands only, as reviewed in Chapter 6 because you get what you pay, so skip most retail pharmacy brands.

Some multivitamins with minerals still don't have therapeutic amounts of certain nutrients for diarrhea, such as zinc, vitamin A, vitamin D, vitamin K2, and calcium. You probably should evaluate your baseline diet to see if you need more of these nutrients. Or, if you know that calcium helps your body overcome diarrhea, you should add those in until you feel better.

Here is a review of the foods with very high amounts of these nutrients to help you sort this out. I'm not talking about moderate amounts of these nutrients. If you have diarrhea, you need the best food sources of these nutrients.

Zinc: Organ meats, shellfish, beef

Vitamin A: Liver, cod liver oil

Vitamin D: Sun exposure in the summer (you need extra supplements of vitamin D the rest of the year in most cases)

Vitamin K2: Natto

Calcium: Yogurt, cheese, broccoli, chia (but poorly absorbed in plant sources)

If you don't currently have access to summer sun or any of these food sources, I recommend supplementing them in addition to the amounts in the multivitamins with minerals. It can't be stressed enough that you should check your vitamin D levels twice yearly and aim for blood levels of around 50ng/ml. Aside from that, there are no good blood tests for the rest of the nutrients because nutrients are stored in your tissues, not your blood. That is why it is important to think about the foods in your diet and whether or not they are truly helping you overcome a deficiency.

I recommend organ meat supplements for additional vitamins and minerals, especially zinc and vitamin A. Alternatively, you can supplement zinc as zinc carnosine at doses of 75–150 mg per day. Vitamin A supplements can be given in doses of around 5000–10,000 IU daily for most adults as a short-term repletion strategy. But, if you have heavy periods or high amounts of inflammation, you can probably continue this dose longer. The key to supplementing vitamin A, as reviewed in Chapter 6, is having adequate vitamin D. Vitamin K2 and vitamin E are also good to add because diarrhea can cause these nutrients to be low.

Case Study: Happy to Have Normal Bowel Movements

Apart from a daily alcoholic drink and coffee, Heather had a healthy diet about 80 percent of the time, drinking herbal tea daily and eating culinary herbs for their anti-inflammatory properties. Yet Heather had frequent bouts of loose stools and eczema.

While technically her diarrhea symptoms were mild, they happened regularly. Her doctor ruled out any other condition, so it was suggested that she take Imodium® to help control the symptoms.

While the Imodium® did stop diarrhea, she noticed that it would constipate her every time she took it. So she decided to see if there were any natural alternatives. We discovered she responded best to taking beef intestines, liver, and stomach supplements using the like-treats-like approach.

She also agreed to stop drinking alcohol, minimize sugar intake, limit gluten, and avoid excess caffeine. Nutritionally, she added vitamin A palmitate and vitamin D3, vitamin K2, broad-spectrum multiple vitamins with minerals, and a spore-based (bacillus) probiotic daily. These supplements helped make up for the losses caused by her routine alcohol intake and eating processed foods.

Heather now only has occasional diarrhea and added the magnesium supplement she knew her body needed. Additionally, her rash nearly disappears after several months of her nutritional regimen.

13

Chapter 13

IBS and SIBO: Curative Answers

Almost half of all visits to GI doctors are because of irritable bowel syndrome symptoms (IBS). However, the scope is much bigger than that because at least 40 percent of people with IBS symptoms don't have a diagnosis of IBS. Additionally, most people with IBS don't seek medical attention at all, so the problem is much bigger than is reported. Because IBS is closely connected to a daunting condition called small intestinal bacterial overgrowth (SIBO), IBS is a condition that needs proper treatment.

In this chapter, learn about what IBS and SIBO are, how to help these conditions with diet, and how to help heal these conditions with supplements and lifestyle changes.

What are IBS and SIBO, and How Are They Related?

Along with abdominal pain symptoms and altered bowel patterns, IBS often has many bodily symptoms. These can include migraine headaches, poor sleep, anxiety, depression, fibromyalgia, or chronic pelvic pain.

There is also a huge overlap with SIBO, and according to the Cleveland Clinic, up to 80 percent of people with IBS have SIBO. So if you have IBS, you can also be safe assuming that it was likely caused by SIBO.

IBS related to SIBO can be aggravated or caused by many other things, including slow gut motility, vitamin and mineral deficiencies, stress, an altered microbiome, gut surgeries, lack of healing foods, etc.

It is important to know that research shows that IBS is often related to a prior gut infection or food poisoning. According to a ground-breaking researcher in IBS, Dr. Tuteja, people who travel abroad have a 50 percent chance of developing IBS.[198]

There are three kinds of IBS, and these are the traditional criteria for diagnosis:

IBS-C: Constipation dominant, with at least 25 percent of stools presenting this way. But differs from chronic constipation because it is usually also accompanied by moderate-to-severe abdominal pain at least three days a month. And it alternates with some bouts of diarrhea and nausea as well.

IBS-D: Diarrhea dominant is essentially like IBS-C, but instead of constipation, you have diarrhea at least 25 percent of the time and constipation less than 25 percent of the time. It also is accompanied by abdominal pain.

IBS-mixed: A combination of constipation and diarrhea accompanied by abdominal pain and discomfort.

SIBO or **small bacterial overgrowth**: This can have any and all of the symptoms listed above but always comes with bloating, especially after meals, and abdominal pain as symptoms, along with altered bowel movements. Otherwise, lean people and overweight people alike feel that their bellies bloat out and feel like they "appear pregnant" even though they aren't. Methane-dominant SIBO typically results in more constipation than not, but SIBO can be just like IBS with diarrhea and constipation.

As you can see, if you have been told you have IBS or SIBO, there is a gray area for diagnosing these conditions using traditional methods. However, new lab tests are available that are 98 percent accurate in detecting IBS. These

---

[198] Tuteja A, Talley N, et al. Development of functional diarrhea, constipation, irritable bowel syndrome, and dyspepsia during and after traveling outside the USA. *Dig Dis Sci.* 2008 Jan;53(1):271–6.

tests are called IBS Smart Tests that measure antibodies called anti-CdtB and anti-vinculin. Because these tests are so newly developed, your doctor or healthcare provider may not yet know about them, but you can encourage them to order this test for you.

For SIBO testing, breath testing is used to diagnose and includes hydrogen breath tests and methane tests. These tests require a skilled practitioner who knows the timing of when to administer these after specific foods are eaten.

Treating IBS and SIBO with Diet

Diet can and should be the cornerstone of helping overcome IBS and SIBO. When you look at conventional texts about treating IBS, there is usually a huge gap related to treating it and looking at the whole person for healing and nourishing the body with food. Rather, there are many don'ts and no mention of actual healing foods and foods and supplements that promote relaxation and motility while restoring the gut microbiome.

When helping people, it is best to take a more holistic approach because at the root of IBS and SIBO are slow gut muscle movements, unwanted bacteria, an altered immune response, vitamin and mineral deficiencies, stress, an altered microbiome, gut barrier disruption, and a lack of healing foods. In other words, there is no single prescription drug that can tackle all of these things. Because even if it is food poisoning or SIBO causing the symptoms, the immune system needs to be bolstered by strengthening the gut and by enhancing immune function so that the issue is more permanently resolved.

Be aware that if you read about SIBO treatment on some websites and in some books, they use protocols that follow a "kill phase," followed by a "healing phase," and then a "recovery phase." Please know that there is no science to this step-by-step process, and biologically speaking, it makes no sense. In fact, it makes much more sense to work on healing to bolster immunity and gut health while simultaneously killing off bad bacteria.

Did You Know . . . You Need to Eat a Healing Diet

I encourage you to closely examine healing foods and supplements to make the most out of your IBS and SIBO treatments. For example, rather than eliminating high FODMAPS foods and taking an antibiotic, why not add healing bone broth, nourishing organ meats, and healing vitamins and minerals like zinc carnosine and magnesium when needed. Why not add in nourishing stews with grass-finished meats, pastured pork, and fish too.

Additionally, try adding more nutrient-rich, microbiome-supporting fats and vegetables and fruits that are easy to digest, such as squash, sweet potatoes, avocado, berries, cooked greens, extra virgin olive oil, coconut oil, and fermented nuts and seeds.

Fats like coconut oil reduce the growth of harmful bacteria in the small bowel while improving nutrient absorption, so it is a very important type of fat to include in a healing diet. Fats, in general, also help lubricate the gut, making bowel movements easier to pass.

For example, extra virgin olive oil is a great tool for reducing constipation, and I recommend having at least 3 tablespoons per day to promote fullness and support healthy bowel movements. If you can't see yourself usually eating this much olive oil, you can have a spoonful or two on its own. Remember, IBS is infection-related, so you need to get the bowels moving so that harmful bacteria can pass- with enough healthy fats to recover. Extra virgin olive oil also provides many polyphenols that support a healthy microbiome.

Another point for healing: don't skimp on protein at meals because protein foods enhance the microbiome, as we reviewed earlier, and protein promotes a feeling of fullness. You should also remove potentially problematic foods such as grains, nightshades, non-fermented dairy, legumes, and added sugars. And as with any gut issues, please don't drink alcohol—it is very toxic to the gut and liver.

Sugar dampens the immune response pretty severely and causes inflammation, so it's a big problem for IBS of any kind. You may feel ok having some rice and corn, but remember, these foods are fairly low in nutrient density, so eat them only if you can't resist the urge. This is a Paleo diet style of eating, which tends to be my favorite because it is the least restrictive.

You likely don't have to eat this way forever, but if you want to heal, I suggest sticking with this diet for at least a month. Then, if bowel movements are going well and you are feeling much better, you can slowly introduce other foods into your diet one at a time, such as nightshade vegetables and other grains and dairy.

Other diet options include:

Intermittent Fasting

This is a very powerful tool for helping IBS. In fact, research shows that it helped reduce seven out of ten IBS symptoms effectively. [199] Also, it is one of the easiest eating strategies to follow if you work your way into it slowly. It helps by dampening inflammation in the gut, helping to restore sleep cycles, improving gut muscle movements via the **migrating motor complex,** and reducing gas and bloating pain. It even helps to reduce chronic pain symptoms! You can combine intermittent fasting with the healing diet as mentioned above but start slow so you are more likely to succeed.

For example, start with eating in a twelve-hour window during the day, such as 6 p.m. to 6 a.m., and gradually decrease the eating window to around eight hours, such as 6 p.m. to 10 a.m. But keep in mind that you don't have to do it all of the time or every day to reap the benefits. I find that using an electrolyte supplement and staying well hydrated during fasting times is very helpful to accept getting used to this eating style. You can find a high-quality electrolyte supplement low in sugar on Fullscript.

---

[199] Kanazawa M, Fukudo S. Effects of fasting therapy on irritable bowel syndrome. *Int J Behav Med.* 2006;13(3):214–20.

Low FODMAP Diet or Low Fermentation Diet

This minimizes fermentable carbohydrates like wheat, cruciferous vegetables, legumes, and fruits like peaches and apples but has no thought of including healing compounds and foods. It allows plenty of inflammatory foods, too, which ironically suppress the immune response.

Keto Diet

Eliminates most carbohydrate-rich foods and encourages more fats like coconut oil, avocados, and extra virgin olive oil. While it may help IBS and SIBO because it eliminates the painful offending foods, there isn't too much focus on diet quality.

Carnivore Diet

This is becoming more and more popular. It is an animal-based diet with little or no plant intake. No research has proven this to be helpful yet. However, many popular social media accounts are recommending it for digestive health, and it has eliminated digestive concerns like IBS for some people. It's pretty restrictive to follow.

Keep in mind that whatever diet pattern you do choose, you can sometimes feel temporarily worse before feeling better due to healing reactions. This usually passes within one week, and you can lessen the healing reaction by adding healing supplements, as we will discuss soon.

Did You Know . . . Treat Yourself with TLC

Additional lifestyle tips for helping overcome IBS and SIBO are making sure that you get enough sleep to bolster your immune system, exercise daily so that you help stimulate the bowels, reduce your stress levels, getting sunshine every day if possible, keeping up with your hydration, and working with an experienced practitioner such as a functional nutritionist or functional medicine doctor.

Supplements to Help Heal the Gut with IBS/SIBO

At the root of IBS and SIBO is often a leaky gut; research indicates that the gut wall is compromised with IBS by measuring a leaky gut protein called zonulin. [200] So supplements that help heal a leaky gut can help reduce IBS symptoms. For example, using probiotics such as *Bifidobacterium longum* helps to reduce zonulin and also reduces inflammation along with a reduction in symptoms of IBS, according to one clinical study.[201]

One more note about supplementation: using a multiple-supplement approach will be more successful than adding one at a time. IBS/SIBO symptoms are rooted in many gut imbalances, not just one. So, for example, adding zinc carnosine, glutamine, multivitamin and minerals, digestive enzymes with bile salts, and bovine colostrum simultaneously is not too many supplements when dealing with challenging IBS. You should read the supplements below to decide what makes the most sense for your body's symptoms. Remember, they all work in different ways, so it makes sense to use several of them as long as you double-check with your healthcare provider.

Organ meats: Especially intestines and liver, will help support like-treats-like in the case of IBS and SIBO. These highly nutritious supplements can replace many other vitamins and minerals if you use them regularly. Many people claim that they tend to heal with organ meats when nothing else has worked. I experience similar benefits.

NAG, or n-acetylglucosamine: This is a beloved supplement for reducing painful GI symptoms in many people, including those with IBS or SIBO. This healing supplement not only helps repair the gut by making protective

---

[200] Fasano A. All disease begins in the (leaky) gut: role of zonulin-mediated gut permeability in the pathogenesis of some chronic inflammatory diseases. *F1000Res.* 2020 Jan 31;9:F1000 Faculty Rev-69.

[201] Serek P, Oleksy-Wawrzyniak M. The Effect of bacterial infections, probiotics and zonulin on intestinal barrier integrity. *Int J Mol Sci.* 2021 Oct 21;22(21):11359.

proteins for the gut lining, but it may also help reduce the stubborn biofilm formation of harmful bacteria, including E. coli.

Zinc carnosine: Blood levels of zinc are lower in people who have IBS-D, and these low levels also are related to a leaky gut. Adding in zinc carnosine may help eradicate some of the unwanted bacteria in the small bowel as well as help heal the intestinal lining. Common doses used in research are 75–150 mg per day of zinc carnosine.[202]

Did You Know . . . Glutamine Is a Healing Powerhouse

Glutamine: As the gut's primary fuel, glutamine helps many digestive disorders, and IBS is no exception. One research study showed that 5 g of glutamine powder three times a day reduced all IBS symptoms, including the severity and normalization of bowel movements, and helped heal the gut wall.[203] In another study, adding glutamine powder to a low FODMAP diet worked better than a low FODMAP diet alone for recovery from IBS symptoms.[204] Personally, I find that you can probably get away with a lower dose than that; try starting at 5 g per day and sip slowly on it. One note of caution: if you have impaired liver function or drink alcohol, check with your doctor before adding glutamine. Alcohol is toxic to the gut, so you should avoid or limit it anyway.

Collagen: Supplements may help heal the gut and are clinically proven to help reduce gut bloating. Daily doses of collagen supplements of 20 g per day are helpful because they help provide healing amino acids for the gut, too, and even promote healthy cholesterol levels.

Multivitamins with minerals: When you have IBS and/or SIBO, the bacteria

---

[202] Hewlings S, Kalman D. A review of zinc-1-carnosine and its positive effects on oral mucositis, taste disorders, and gastrointestinal disorders. *Nutrients*. 2020 Feb 29;12(3):665.

[203] Zhou Q, Verne M, et al. Randomised placebo-controlled trial of dietary glutamine supplements for postinfectious irritable bowel syndrome. *Gut*. 2019 Jun;68(6):996–1002.

[204] Rastgoo S, Ebrahimi-Daryani N, et al. Glutamine supplementation enhances the effects of a low FODMAP diet in irritable bowel syndrome management. *Front Nutr*. 2021 Dec 16;8:746703. doi: 10.3389/fnut.2021.746703. PMID: 34977110; PMCID: PMC8716871.

in the small bowel gobble up your body's vitamins and minerals. These harmful bacteria rob you. So it makes sense to add in a good multivitamin with minerals and/or add in organ meat supplements. I've had clients who I coaxed into adding multivitamins and mineral supplements, and it was the only thing that eased some of their IBS symptoms, such as nausea. By replenishing your vitamins, you are also bolstering your immune system to fight off unwanted bacteria in the small bowel, so it is a win-win.

Bovine colostrum: This can help gobble up unwanted SIBO-type bacteria while helping to heal the gut wall and reduce leaky gut. Studies of athletes using bovine colostrum confirm that it helps heal the gut lining. Using 1 teaspoon a day and increasing as tolerated to 1 tablespoon per day is a common dose of this supplement that helps with many aspects of health. I personally won't live without my 1 tablespoon per day. You must avoid bovine colostrum if you have a milk allergy, but you can try IgG, which I will explain next.

IgG (Immunoglobulin G): This a supplement that helps reduce diarrhea-predominant IBS symptoms, according to several clinical studies. It is dairy-free, and a typical dose is 5 g per day of IgG, available on Fullscript (see page 306 for recommendations).

Omega-3 fats: People with IBS tend to have higher levels of inflammatory fats in their blood, called omega-6 fats, while they have reduced omega-3 anti-inflammatory levels. The best way to supplement omega-3 fats is by using cod liver oil, as reviewed in Chapter 7. This is because cod liver oil is best absorbed when it has healing vitamin A.

Digestive enzymes: These are perhaps one of the most critical supplements to take to reduce symptoms of IBS, and they also help your body absorb the food you eat better. They are very helpful for reducing gas and bloating. They also have anti-inflammatory effects on their own. Just take a broad-spectrum enzyme supplement, as reviewed in Chapter 7, and take it with each meal for the best results. Adding a Fodzyme enzyme may also help a lot.

Melatonin: A common supplement that, interestingly, may help IBS symptoms. In fact, all human studies have consistently shown a reduction in abdominal pain with melatonin use, and some showed improvement in quality of life in people with IBS. Melatonin may help improve gut muscle movements, provides natural pain relief, and promotes improved sleep quality, all of which help improve gut health. For IBS, doses of 3–6 mg per day are effective.

Butyrate: A substance that fuels intestinal cells and is considered a postbiotic, as discussed in Chapter 8. New research in a large-scale study shows that butyrate at 150 mg twice daily reduces IBS symptoms when given over twelve weeks. It significantly reduced gas, diarrhea, constipation, bowel urgency, nausea, and vomiting in people with IBS.[205]

Probiotics: These are very helpful in managing most IBS symptoms and should be considered a cornerstone of therapy and healing for IBS. They are even proven to help manage SIBO too. But, as reviewed previously, your microbiome is unique, so the strains that help you the most may take some trial and error. Based on previous research, a good place to start is by using Bacillus or soil-based strains first. [206] [207]Another excellent choice is Saccharomyces boulardii. Clinical studies also show the benefits of Bifidobacterium, but you will need higher doses of 10–20 billion CFUs if you go with these types of probiotics.

Bile salts: This helps reduce SIBO symptoms and reduces methane-producing bacteria. In fact, people with SIBO and functional dyspepsia typically don't make enough bile at mealtimes. Bile acids are generally helpful for absorbing fats, vitamins, and minerals. Research using it used 100 mg of bile salts daily with meals.

Activated charcoal: Helps to rid the body of toxins and gas and, fascinatingly, is more effective than antibiotic treatment for SIBO symptoms,

---

[205] Lewandowski K, Kaniewska M, et al. The effectiveness of microencapsulated sodium butyrate at reducing symptoms in patients with irritable bowel syndrome. *Prz Gastroenterol.* 2022;17(1):28–34.

[206] Gabrielli M, Lauritano E, et al. Bacillus clausii as a treatment of small intestinal bacterial overgrowth. *Am J Gastroenterol.* 2009 May;104(5):1327–8.

[207] Khalighi A, Khalighi M, et al. Evaluating the efficacy of probiotic on treatment in patients with small intestinal bacterial overgrowth (SIBO)—a pilot study. *Indian J Med Res.* 2014 Nov;140(5):604–8.

according to research. [208] It is also effective in helping reduce diarrhea symptoms. One more thing: it may even help heal a leaky gut, which is a good thing. Generally speaking, it is best to take activated charcoal on an empty stomach and away from most medications and other supplements because it binds to so many things. A good starting dose is 500-1000 mg per day. For more information, read my blog post about coconut charcoal here: https://thehealthyrd.com/surprising-coconut-charcoal-benefits-for-gut-health-and-more/

Vitamin D3: Because vitamin D helps to make natural anti-microbial and boost both innate and adaptive immunity, you must test your vitamin D levels and aim for a blood level of 50 ng/ml or so by supplementing vitamin D3 to get to that level. Vitamin D3 reduces IBS severity, helps you to have a healthy microbiome, and kills unwanted bacteria. Talk about triple-pronged therapy! There is no one-size-fits-all approach to dosing. Some people need 2,000 IU per day, while others need over 10,000 IU per day. That is why it is extra important that you test levels and repeat.

Caprylic acid: This is an important MCT oil supplement for some people with IBS and SIBO because it helps reduce candida overgrowth and bacterial overgrowth and reduces bacterial biofilms, which are common issues with these conditions. Caprylic acid is very potent, so a little goes a long way, and it is best to start with a teaspoon a day in a sipped beverage rather than gulped. This supplement is also a very effective remedy for constipation, but start low and slow.

Get Your Bowels Moving (or Slow Them Down)

For most people with IBS-C or SIBO, regulating the bowels is the most important factor because it reduces the chances that bacteria grow where they aren't supposed to grow in the small intestine. If the supplements listed above aren't adequate to regulate your bowels, there are other remedies you

[208] Hübner W, Moser E. Charcoal tablets in the treatment of patients with irritable bowel syndrome. *Adv Ther.* 2002 Sep–Oct;19(5):245–52.

can try. This section gives you remedies for both sluggish bowels and for people with too frequent bowel movements as well.

Sluggish Bowels (IBS-C) remedies

Very similar to the remedies discussed in Chapter 11 for constipation, constipation remedies can be all-natural and helpful for helping IBS-C. Also, remember that the biggest distinction between chronic constipation and IBS-C is that IBS-C comes with abdominal pain at least three days a month, whereas chronic constipation does not.

Magnesium

So if the healing supplements listed above aren't enough to accomplish soft and easy-to-pass daily bowel movements, I recommend trying magnesium until you have a bowel movement daily. Then, you should continue daily magnesium to keep up with regular stools. Good magnesium choices for IBS-C are magnesium citrate and magnesium oxide powders or capsules. Just start with the dose suggested on the product label you buy.

Betaine HCL

If your IBS-C is accompanied by indigestion and bloating, you may also want to add some apple cider vinegar with the mother into your diet or try adding betaine HCL with mealtimes. This is because a lack of stomach acid can create many downstream issues in the gut, even constipation due to indigestion. Betaine HCL often also comes with pepsin, which is good because it helps the body break down protein. Be sure not to confuse Betaine HCL with betaine anhydrous, as they are two different supplements. Low stomach acid also frequently contributes to SIBO, which happens in most people with IBS-C. However, if you take betaine HCL and find any stomach discomfort, you shouldn't take it.

Prebiotic Fiber

For IBS, fiber can be very tricky to supplement, but in some cases, it can be quite beneficial. Fibers such as acacia fiber, followed by guar gum, beta-glucan, and psyllium, are good prebiotic fibers that can be slowly introduced to the diet to help add bulk to the stool, which can reduce IBS-diarrhea symptoms as well as IBS-constipation symptoms. Some people also do great with chicory fiber or inulin, but this one needs a slow introduction for many because it can ramp up gas and bloat. A good rule of thumb is to start with around 2–3 g of prebiotic fiber per day. If this goes well, increase the dose to twice that amount after 1 week. But, if you feel any symptoms worsen, you should back off. Also, the most important thing you should do is to hydrate well while adding in prebiotic fibers, or they can definitely worsen constipation symptoms by solidifying the stool too much.

Other Herbal Remedies

Artichoke leaf extract: is another useful herbal therapy for people with IBS because it helps normalize bowel patterns and reduces dyspepsia symptoms. Not only that, artichoke leaf extract is good for keeping the liver and biliary tract healthy as well. It's a very safe supplement; people eat artichoke leaves as food, after all. Still, if you are allergic to it, you should avoid it. Common doses of artichoke leaf extract vary from 600–800 mg per day.

Senna: is a plant with natural laxative properties and is effective in helping treat constipation. It is also well-tolerated, and contrary to dogmatic thinking, it is not addictive or habit-forming. In fact, research shows that it is more effective than Miralax (polyethylene glycol) for constipation, with fewer side effects than drug therapy.[209] And compared to conventional laxatives, senna also helps reduce inflammatory compounds and promotes

---

[209] Santos-Jasso K, Arredondo-García J, et al. Effectiveness of senna vs polyethylene glycol as laxative therapy in children with constipation related to anorectal malformation. *J Pediatr Surg.* 2017 Jan;52(1):84–8.

normal muscle movements of the intestine. You can either sip on senna tea or use senna capsules which are typically in doses of around 400 mg per capsule. Most people find it gentle with little to no side effects at all.

Caraway and Peppermint: the combination of caraway and peppermint are often very effective for many gut conditions, and IBS is no exception. For example, these two herbs significantly reduced IBS-associated symptoms, including pain, gas, diarrhea, fullness, and feelings of pressure. The product used in research is called Menthacarin, but this exact product is not available commercially. [210] See page 305 for a similar product on Fullscript; a typical dosage is 1 gel cap per day.

Herbal Therapies for IBS and SIBO

Herbal therapies can be very helpful with just about every aspect of IBS and SIBO. While this is a partial list of herbs, it is a good start for anyone suffering from these conditions. Remember that I am giving you the clinical indications research has shown for these particular herbs. [211] And also, keep in mind that they actually can work better than conventional medicines too.

Aloe vera: Aloe is clinically proven to help IBS symptoms and makes the most sense to be used in people who struggle with constipation-predominant IBS. It can help stimulate intestinal muscle movements and to pull water towards it, allowing for easier bowel movements. Like many herbs, it is also naturally anti-inflammatory. What is surprising, according to research, is that it is also helpful for IBS-diarrhea-predominant symptoms like pain. [212] Using aloe is cheap, safe, and readily available in most retail pharmacies.

[210] Madisch A, Miehlke S, et al. Effectiveness of Menthacarin on symptoms of irritable bowel syndrome. *Wien Med Wochenschr.* 2019 Apr;169(5–6):149–55.

[211] Hawrelak J, Wohlmuth H, et al. Western herbal medicines in the treatment of irritable bowel syndrome: A systematic review and meta-analysis. *Complement Ther Med.* 2020 Jan;48:102233.

[212] Hong S, Chun J, et al. Aloe vera is effective and safe in short-term treatment of irritable bowel syndrome: A systematic review and meta-analysis. J *Neurogastroenterol Motil.* 2018 Oct 1;24(4):528–35.

However, it is still best to go with a reputable brand, and you can find those on Fullscript. People use both capsules and aloe vera juice successfully, and the dose of aloe juice is typically 2 oz or 1 capsule per day.

Dysbiocide and FC Cidal: For people who struggle with SIBO, herbal therapies are often surprisingly more effective than antibiotics and, in one study, were better at controlling SIBO than antibiotics. In this study, they used either Dysbiocide and FC Cidal herbal therapies or Candibactin-AR and Candibactin-BR of 2 capsules twice daily each for four weeks.[213] Interestingly, the herbal therapies also had fewer side effects than the antibiotics group. You must get these from a reputable herbal dispensary at your local natural health food store or through Fullscript. I recommend seeing a knowledgeable functional medicine doctor if you want to try this kind of remedy.

Ginger and Peppermint: A combination of ginger and peppermint improves symptoms of IBS in people already receiving conventional treatments for IBS. The dose used in the clinical trial was 730 mg per day for thirty days. Both ginger and peppermint are generally considered safe too. Because it is difficult to find this exact combination as a supplement, you should know that the research trial used peppermint oil at 240 mg with 40 percent menthol, 1.5 percent limonene, and 50 mg of ginger oil with standardized 14 percent gingerol.[214] See page 306 for recommendations.

Iberogast: A herbal formulation of nine herbs, as reviewed in Chapter 7, has multiple actions on IBS, including normalizing gut muscle movements, reducing inflammation, regulating gastric secretions, and improving the microbiome. It is also very well-tolerated by most people. This supplement is harder to find because it is an Australian product, but it is available on Amazon. Please note that it does contain licorice root, so you should consult with your healthcare provider before taking this product.

Turmeric: Because turmeric is a potent anti-inflammatory spice, it may

---

[213] Chedid V, Dhalla S, et al. Herbal therapy is equivalent to rifaximin for the treatment of small intestinal bacterial overgrowth. *Glob Adv Health Med.* 2014 May;3(3):16–24.

[214] Ivashkin V, Kudryavtseva A, et al. Efficacy and safety of a food supplement with standardized menthol, limonene, and gingerol content in patients with irritable bowel syndrome: A double-blind, randomized, placebo-controlled trial. *PLoS One.* 2022 Jun 15;17(6):e0263880.

help ease some symptoms of IBS. However, there isn't much robust research to prove this. But one small study found that when turmeric was combined with boswellia, 500 mg a day total, along with a low FODMAP diet, symptoms of SIBO were reduced more than just a low FODMAP diet alone. [215] Another study showed that 500 mg of turmeric as Curcugen™ reduced digestive symptoms of IBS.[216] Still, turmeric can be a fairly common intolerance and upsetting to some people's digestive tracts, so just be sure to stop taking it if you feel worse. Make sure to take turmeric with a substantial meal with fat for the best absorption. Turmeric is related to ginger, so it has similar gut-enhancing effects, which include a reduction in harmful bacteria, reduced pain, and an improved microbiome. See page 308 for recommendations.

Other Very Useful Herbs for IBS and SIBO include:

Garlic (as stabilized allicin): Reduces the growth of harmful bacteria and is often used as part of herbal antimicrobial regimens for SIBO. It helps kill off bad bacteria due to infections and SIBO. Many people use it as a general immune support and to help lower blood pressure. The good thing about this form of garlic is that it is free of **FODMAPS,** which can irritate IBS symptoms. See page 306 for recommendations.

Quercetin: It helps to promote bowel regularity and dampens inflammation, so it could be a helpful antioxidant supplement to add if you have IBS and/or SIBO.

Fennel seeds: Useful in IBS and SIBO because it helps to regulate the bowels and may help reduce infectious types of diarrhea.

Coriander: Helps to reduce abdominal bloating and discomfort in people with IBS, and it's great added to almost any kind of food. It isn't readily available as a supplement, so you can make tea if you don't want to add it to

---

[215] Giacosa A, Riva A, et al. Beneficial effects on abdominal bloating with an innovative food-grade formulation of curcuma longa and Boswellia serrata extracts in subjects with irritable bowel syndrome and small bowel dysbiosis. *Nutrients.* 2022 Jan 18;14(3):416

[216] Lopresti A, Smith S, et al. Efficacy of a curcumin extract (Curcugen™) on gastrointestinal symptoms and intestinal microbiota in adults with self-reported digestive complaints: A randomised, double-blind, placebo-controlled study. *BMC Complement Med Ther.* 2021 Jan 21;21(1):40.

cooking.

Milk Thistle: Reduces gas and bloating and even helps balance the microbiome, so it is a gentle and safe approach for people with IBS and SIBO. You can get milk thistle tea or capsules. See page 307 for recommendations.

Oregano: A potent antimicrobial herb that also helps boost immune function while dampening inflammation. See page 307 for recommendations.

Thyme: Helps support healthy immunity and reduces harmful bacteria, as in SIBO. You can make thyme tea or get a thyme tincture. See page 308 for recommendations.

Case Study: Fasting and a Healing Regimen Eradicates SIBO and IBS Symptoms

Anne had just about every gut symptom you could imagine—gas, pain, bloating, heartburn, constipation, but also occasional diarrhea. What's worse, every time she ate, she bloated.

Her issues started with a gut infection while traveling to South America and worsened after her abdominal surgery. The impaired gut muscle movements result in constipation. She was also vegan for a while, which seemed to only make everything feel worse. In the end, all of these things contributed to her having IBS and SIBO as diagnosed by hydrogen breath test and methane breath test.

She had tried taking antibiotics and a course of natural herbal antibiotics for her SIBO with some success, but her symptoms returned within a month of ending these medications.

To help stimulate normal muscle movements of her gut, she agreed to try intermittent fasting for sixteen hours on most days by eating dinner at 6 p.m. and then not eating again until 10 a.m. This regimen was in addition to eating a healing diet.

To help heal her gut, she started a short-term (two-week) regimen of intensive healing supplements. For the healing regimen, she added a broad-spectrum natural multivitamin with minerals, an IgG supplement, vitamin A palmitate and D3 with vitamin K2, melatonin, magnesium, digestive enzymes, glutamine powder, and the probiotic Saccharomyces boulardii.

To address the SIBO and constipation, she used an oregano gel cap three times daily, Allimax® garlic, and charcoal supplements with meals for a month. She also took senna capsules for constipation.

After a month, she was finally feeling much better without a return of major symptoms, so we switched her to a daily spore-based probiotic but continued with her digestive enzymes, multivitamin, and healing diet. Now, her constipation and digestive symptoms are much less frequent, and she only takes oregano and charcoal capsules when she feels gas and bloating taking over. The most important part of feeling better, she believed, was working on healing her gut and keeping her bowels moving with magnesium, senna, and oregano.

14

Chapter 14

Inflammatory Bowel Disease: An Alternative Therapy

Inflammatory bowel diseases (IBD) are some of the most daunting gut disorders because they can severely affect the quality of life and substantially increase the risk of other diseases like cancer. Interestingly, countries with a lot of poverty have much lower rates of inflammatory bowel diseases, such as Mexico, Africa, and most of South America. The United States has the highest rates of inflammatory bowel disease, with around 252 to 439 cases per 100,000 people having one of these conditions, according to *The Lancet.*[217]

This all points to the fact that industrialized foods and modern lifestyles increase the likelihood of getting one of these miserable conditions. And Big Food and even some pharmaceuticals increase the risk. Drugs like ibuprofen, antibiotics, birth control, anti-rejection drugs, and even food additives like sodium phosphate are related to an increased risk of IBD.

In mainstream medical journals and the media, there is little mention of nutritional therapies and natural approaches for these challenging condi-

---

[217] GBD 2017 Inflammatory Bowel Disease Collaborators. The global, regional, and national burden of inflammatory bowel disease in 195 countries and territories, 1990–2017: A systematic analysis for the global burden of disease study 2017. Lancet Gastroenterol Hepatol. 2020 Jan;5(1):17–30.

tions. And yet most likely, at the root of these conditions is a lack of healing foods and a poor lifestyle. Many peer-reviewed research publications now show the benefits of various eating patterns and supplements in helping to manage these conditions.[218] [219] [220] [221] [222] Still, they lack the attention of mainstream media and medicine because there is no money to be gained from it.

Conventional treatment of IBD includes corticosteroids, biological drugs, and immunosuppressants. Sadly, these drugs have serious long-term risks, such as increased cancer risk, bone fractures, and serious infections.[223] While sometimes needed, these medications don't get to the root of the problem, which is often how we nourish our gut.

In this chapter, you will learn about the different types of inflammatory bowel diseases, diet strategies, and supplements that can help reduce the symptoms and severity of these conditions.

What is Inflammatory Bowel Disease?

Inflammatory bowel diseases aren't one, but many conditions related to high inflammation in the gut. The most common inflammatory bowel diseases are Crohn's, ulcerative, and microscopic colitis.

Crohn's disease affects the small and large intestines, while ulcerative

[218] Shafiee N, Manaf Z, et al. Anti-inflammatory diet and inflammatory bowel disease: what clinicians and patients should know? *Intest Res.* 2021 Apr;19(2):171–85.

[219] Choi Y, Kraft N, et al. Fructose intolerance in IBS and utility of fructose-restricted diet. *J Clin Gastroenterol.* 2008 Mar;42(3):233–8.

[220] Konijeti G, Kim N, et al. Efficacy of the autoimmune protocol diet for inflammatory bowel disease. *Inflamm Bowel Dis.* 2017 Nov;23(11):2054–60.

[221] Weaver K, Herfarth H. Gluten-free diet in IBD: Time for a recommendation? *Mol Nutr Food Res.* 2021 Mar;65(5):e1901274.

[222] Herfarth H, Martin C, et al. Prevalence of a gluten-free diet and improvement of clinical symptoms in patients with inflammatory bowel diseases. *Inflamm Bowel Dis.* 2014 Jul;20(7):1194–7.

[223] Buchman A. Side effects of corticosteroid therapy. *J Clin Gastroenterol.* 2001 Oct;33(4):289–94.

colitis is usually limited to the large intestine. Microscopic colitis is not visible with a colonoscopy but can be detected with a microscope. This type of colitis includes collagenous and lymphocytic colitis, which are very similar. Regardless of the name or form, they are related to inflammation and imbalances in the gut's immune system. Due to the inflammation, your body doesn't absorb nutrients well, and there is a lack of digestive enzymes, especially with Crohn's disease. But because food and supplements can directly affect both of these positively or negatively, there is a lot of self-care that you can do to improve your wellbeing if you have any type of inflammatory bowel disease.

While celiac disease, or gluten-sensitive enteropathy, isn't technically an inflammatory bowel disease, some of the same principles apply, so we will also discuss this condition here.

Symptoms are fairly similar to IBS and can include diarrhea, abdominal pain, fatigue, cramping, unintentional weight loss, malnutrition, blood in the stool, and anemia. The condition is usually diagnosed by endoscopy, stool tests, and various blood tests.

Did You Know . . . When to Seek Help

If you have been diagnosed with inflammatory bowel disease, you most certainly have been to the doctor to determine its diagnosis. But emergent care is sometimes needed, especially if you have an increased frequency of bowel movements which can put you at risk for dehydration and electrolyte disturbances. Also, it is important to seek help immediately if you have blood in your stool or severe abdominal pain.

Diet Strategies for IBD

There is an undeniable link between foods and inflammatory bowel disease. For example, people with celiac disease, where gluten foods are the main culprit, are nine times more likely to have inflammatory bowel disease than people who do not. And you don't have to have celiac disease to have a sensitivity to gluten with IBD, either. Of those with IBD who attempt a gluten-free diet, 56 percent feel less bloating, 46 percent have less diarrhea, 41 percent have less pain, and 38 percent have remission compared to those who don't. Talk about a beneficial and risk-free intervention to try.

For this reason, I highly recommend following a gluten-free diet if you have any type of IBD. Gluten is found in almost all processed foods, too, so by eliminating junk foods, you are already halfway to reducing inflammation. Then, you should also try to avoid wheat, rye, and barley, including beer, pasta, bread, breading, and baked goods. Gluten-free alternatives are usually very tasty such as gluten-free pasta and rice, fermented quinoa, and gluten-free oats-these work as staples if needed. However, rather than eating a bunch of gluten-free fillers, it is best to focus on healing foods, such as bone broth, grass-fed meats, organ meats, wild-caught fish, root vegetables, extra virgin olive oil, and fermented foods if possible. In other words, prioritize healing proteins and fats, and most other things will fall into place.

This reflects an autoimmune protocol diet, which eliminates major food sensitivities like most grains, legumes, nightshades, dairy, eggs, coffee, alcohol, nuts and seeds, refined/processed sugars, oils, and food additives. An autoimmune protocol diet may indeed be a very effective approach to helping with IBD; one study found that this diet regimen reduced gut inflammatory markers called fecal calprotectin, people had an almost five-fold improvement in gut symptoms, 71 percent of people had achieved remission, and they also had improvements in endoscopic scores. [224]

If you are new to the idea of an autoimmune protocol, it is a Paleo style of eating, and you can find many cookbooks and books about how to follow this style of eating. There are also autoimmune protocol cookbooks as well. The full elimination of foods is temporary as well; foods after a few months can slowly be reintroduced as tolerated, one at a time, once the body has healed. Dr. Terry Wahls also proved that the autoimmune protocol can be as nutritious or more nutritious than the food recommended by the US dietary

---

[224] Konijeti G, Kim N, et al. Efficacy of the autoimmune protocol diet for inflammatory bowel disease. *Inflamm Bowel Dis.* 2017 Nov;23(11):2054–60.

guidelines. [225]

Also, at least a third of people with IBD have fructose intolerance. Foods that are VERY high in fructose are sodas, grape juice, cranberry juice cocktail, and sweet tea. Natural foods like jackfruit, apples, grapes, pears, raisins, and blueberries are also high. Sadly, honey also has a fairly high amount of fructose as well. Luckily natural maple syrup is quite low in fructose, so that can be a nice sweetener alternative.

Common sense also applies. If you know you react to any food, you should avoid it, too, until you can heal your gut. This can include "healthy" foods like many vegetables. Elimination isn't forever, but eating a healing diet and reducing inflammation can make your tolerance to offending foods improve over time. Healing supplements can be a godsend, too, and we will get into those next.

Early research even shows promise for using a **ketogenic diet** for colitis because it may improve gut barrier function, reduce inflammation, and improve the microbiome compared to a normal carbohydrate diet. [226] [227]However, because we are all unique, this plan is not for everyone, and it takes a lot of know-how and extreme commitment. Even with a keto diet, there can be a lot of gaps in nutrients, and the quality of foods and nutrients needs to be considered.

The Healing Supplement Combination

With IBD conditions, the key thing to work on is nourishing and healing. By healing, you help stop inflammatory compounds from entering your bloodstream. And because gut cells reproduce every five days, the potential

---

[225] Konijeti G, Kim N, et al. Efficacy of the autoimmune protocol diet for inflammatory bowel disease. *Inflamm Bowel Dis.* 2017 Nov;23(11):2054–60.

[226] Chenard C, Rubenstein L, et al. Nutrient composition comparison between a modified paleolithic diet for multiple sclerosis and the recommended healthy U.S.-style eating pattern. *Nutrients.* 2019 Mar 1;11(3):537.

[227] Kong C, Yan X, et al. Ketogenic diet alleviates colitis by reduction of colonic group 3 innate lymphoid cells through altering gut microbiome. *Sig Transduct Target Ther.* 2021: 6, 154.

to heal is real, even with daunting conditions like IBD. I suggest starting with several of these at a time because the more healing compounds you can bathe your gut cells, the quicker you may feel better.

For example, having organ meats, collagen, digestive enzymes, vitamin D and K2, and cod liver oil is a good starting point. Still, it's good to review your supplement regimen with your healthcare provider, that hopefully is well-versed in the topic of nutrition, such as a functional medicine doctor or a functional nutritionist.

It is extremely unlikely that you will get too many nutrients because people with IBD are almost always behind the game in nutrients. Supplementation for two weeks may be enough of these whole food compounds to get you well on your way to healing if you also pay close attention to your diet. This chapter reverts Chapter 7 in many ways because IBD requires most healing compounds.

Cod liver oil: There have been many studies that show that fish oil helps reduce symptoms of ulcerative colitis. But it stands to reason that cod liver oil would help a lot more because it absorbs better and can contain healing amounts of vitamin A. Most people can stand to have more vitamin A and more omega-3s, so I do recommend adding cod liver oil daily as long as you choose brands that contain natural vitamin A in them (see page 305 for recommendations).

Vitamin D: It isn't a coincidence that countries with more poverty are often in warmer climates. This is perhaps partly why some countries like Mexico have fewer cases of inflammatory bowel diseases. Research shows that vitamin D is very helpful for people with IBD. For example, vitamin D supplementation reduces the severity of symptoms of ulcerative colitis in people receiving higher amounts of vitamin D. People with low vitamin D levels are also more likely to get Crohn's disease and microscopic colitis celiac disease in the first place.

Organ meats: These are indispensable nutritionally speaking and have been used for thousands of years for their healing benefits. Good choices of organ meats are reviewed in Chapter 7, and I highly recommend adding grass-fed beef intestines and grass-fed beef liver and spleen if you have colitis. I recommend taking two of each with meals for a few weeks to see if you feel better. Organ meats contain powerful building blocks and bio directors to their own specific tissues (like treats like) along with high amounts of healing collagen, vitamins, and minerals.

Collagen: People who suffer from inflammatory bowel diseases often have low collagen levels, so using collagen-rich foods or collagen supplements makes a lot of sense. Collagen helps the body make bile, helps heal the gut lining, and even reduces symptoms of daunting conditions like asthma. People with IBD often have low bone density, and collagen research shows it helps reduce bone loss. [228] [229]Bone broth is a great source of collagen, so I encourage you to cook with it and add it to soups, stews, and main dishes.

NAG: This is powerfully healing and dramatically reduces abdominal pain in people with gut issues like IBD. For example, in children with severe Crohn's disease, NAG was given. It reduced the need for abdominal surgery, reduced symptoms of Crohn's, and even reduced inflammation, as shown on the biopsy, according to a small study.[230] NAG is an amino acid supplement that is non-toxic and safe, so it's definitely worth a try. The only caution is that because it is derived from shellfish, you may need to avoid using it if you have a shellfish allergy.

Zinc carnosine: Zinc, in general, is critical for healing and repair and has over 300 functions in the body. But when zinc is combined with the amino acids in carnosine, it is extra healing for the gut. Zinc deficiency is common in people with IBD, and low zinc levels are linked to worse outcomes. One study showed that by giving zinc carnosine enemas one time and 71 percent achieved remission of their ulcerative colitis compared to only 10 percent

[228]Ramadass S, Jabaris S, et al. Type I collagen and its daughter peptides for targeting mucosal healing in ulcerative colitis: A new treatment strategy. *Eur J Pharm Sci.* 2016 Aug 25;91:216–24.

[229]Daneault A, Prawitt J, et al. Biological effect of hydrolyzed collagen on bone metabolism. *Crit Rev Food Sci Nutr.* 2017 Jun 13;57(9):1922–37.

[230]Salvatore S, Heuschkel R, et al. A pilot study of N-acetyl glucosamine, a nutritional substrate for glycosaminoglycan synthesis, in paediatric chronic inflammatory bowel disease. *Aliment Pharmacol Ther.* 2000 Dec;14(12):1567–79.

in the placebo group. [231] It is also used as a dietary supplement, and typical doses are 75 mg given twice daily.

Bovine colostrum: This holds much potential for helping IBD because it can dampen inflammation, heal gut cells, and help with regeneration among early studies. It helps heal a leaky gut and reduces diarrhea episodes in the general population. Strangely enough, the only studies with IBD specifically gave colostrum as an enema, and given this way, it reduced IBD symptoms. Just make sure to avoid it if you have a true milk allergy. Start with 1 teaspoon of bovine colostrum powder and mix it with water. Slowly increase this dose to 1–2 tablespoons a week as tolerated.

Butyrate: Crohn's disease is challenging to treat, but butyrate may help. According to one small study, butyrate helped 69 percent of people, and 53 percent had remission of symptoms. [232] Considering that butyrate is very safe and well-tolerated, it makes sense that it could help you if you have IBD and may even be helpful if you have celiac disease. Foods can increase the production of butyrate, such as soluble fiber foods, but these foods can be problematic for some people with IBD. Refer back to the fiber section in Chapter 7 for more information.

IGG: Helps reduce the frequency of diarrhea in people with IBD conditions, according to one study.[233] It works by gobbling up harmful microbes and helping heal the gut. Of note, it is also a component in bovine colostrum too. Research indicates that it can take up to twelve weeks to work, but almost three times as many people had clinical improvement in their IBD symptoms after using IgG supplements compared to those who did not. IgG supplements are also likely helpful for people with celiac disease because it helps to heal the gut, and celiac disease is more than a gluten problem-it is

[231] Itagaki M, Saruta M, et al. Efficacy of zinc-carnosine chelate compound, Polaprezinc, enemas in patients with ulcerative colitis. *Scand J Gastroenterol.* 2014 Feb;49(2):164–72.

[232] Di Sabatino A, Morera R, et al. Oral butyrate for mildly to moderately active Crohn's disease. *Aliment Pharmacol Ther.* 2005 Nov 1;22(9):789–94. doi: 10.1111/j.1365-2036.2005.02639.x. PMID: 16225487.

[233] Karimi S, Tabataba-vakili S, et al. The effects of two vitamin D regimens on ulcerative colitis activity index, quality of life and oxidant/anti-oxidant status. *Nutr J.* 2019;18, 16.

an absorption problem too.[234]

Glutamine: This may help speed up the healing of the gut lining for people following a healing diet. It is also likely helpful for people who have celiac disease. On its own, it may not help that much if you are eating a standard American diet. Remember that the research around glutamine is messy: they give it in many forms and doses but tend to ignore the baseline diet. This means that the research is inconclusive about it. However, there are clear benefits for glutamine, helping improve the microbiome and helping to reduce leaky gut in conditions like Crohn's disease, ulcerative colitis, and even celiac disease. A typical starting dose is 5 g daily, and I recommend sipping it slowly. Remember, if you have liver disease, you should avoid using glutamine powder.

Digestive Enzymes: Pancreatic disease and IBD are linked, so people with IBD may not make enough pancreatic enzymes to support digestive function. The other issue with IBD is that the intestinal wall is inflamed, which likely means fewer enzymes are made along the intestinal wall. Poor absorption of nutrients is given with Crohn's, so it is yet another reason to consider adding digestive enzymes because they help you absorb food better. Although no clinical studies have been conducted to see if digestive enzymes will help IBD, common sense suggests that they will help because they help reduce bloating and diarrhea symptoms for people in general. They also can help reduce inflammation in the gut.

Probiotics: These hold a lot of promise for helping people with IBD, especially ulcerative colitis. One of the root causes of many bowel diseases is imbalances in bacteria, and IBD is no exception. Especially useful strains seem to be *Bacillus* strains and *Saccharomyces boulardii*. However, as reviewed previously, your individual tolerance for probiotics may vary, so trial and error may be needed.

Acacia fiber: Acacia fiber is a gentle choice to add when your IBD symptoms aren't active because it is less irritating than other types. I recommend

---

[234] Ulfman L, Leusen J, et al. Effects of bovine immunoglobulins on immune function, allergy, and infection. *Front Nutr.* 2018 Jun 22;5:52.

starting with half the dose recommended on your supplement label to see how you tolerate it. Adding soluble fiber like acacia fiber can increase the microbiome's health, and it can also help fuel the gut lining by making butyrate. Keep in mind that the only research that supports using fiber for IBD is preliminary, so try it with caution and discontinue it if you have any side effects. One study also used beta-glucan and saw improved IBD symptoms; they combined it with digestive enzymes.[235] Another good option for naturally adding fiber is beetroot supplements or pectin fiber. Some research even shows that psyllium fiber is helpful for people who struggle with ulcerative colitis.[236]

Herbal Remedies for IBD

When it comes to herbs that may help with IBD symptoms, there are too many to count that may help. This is because of the entourage effect of herbs and their synergistic effects as well as you may recall from Chapter 7.

While research continues to lag behind traditional use, that doesn't mean a lack of benefits. Herbs have anti-inflammatory, calming, microbiome-balancing effects, and more. You will be hard-pressed to wait for studies because the funneling of resources in research almost exclusively goes to Big Pharma. Still, some research points to the benefits of herbs, and here are ones that hold a lot of promise for helping your symptoms if you have any kind of IBD. [237]

[235] Spagnuolo R, Cosco C, et al. Beta-glucan, inositol and digestive enzymes improve quality of life of patients with inflammatory bowel disease and irritable bowel syndrome. *Eur Rev Med Pharmacol Sci.* 2017 Jun;21(2 Suppl):102–7.

[236] Fernández-Bañares F, Hinojosa J, et al. Randomized clinical trial of Plantago ovata seeds (dietary fiber) as compared with mesalamine in maintaining remission in ulcerative colitis. Spanish Group for the Study of Crohn's Disease and Ulcerative Colitis (GETECCU). *Am J Gastroenterol.* 1999 Feb;94(2):427–33.

[237] Holleran G, Scaldaferri F, et al. Herbal medicinal products for inflammatory bowel disease: A focus on those assessed in double-blind randomised controlled trials. *Phytother Res.* 2020 Jan;34(1):77–93.

Cannabis: An anti-inflammatory, so it makes sense that it would help IBD conditions. One study showed that people with IBD using cannabis with THC benefitted 90 percent of patients compared to a placebo, and 45 percent had remission of IBS with cannabis use compared to 10 percent getting a placebo. [238] In other words, cannabis is very helpful, but CBD isn't enough; you need the full flowering cannabis plant with THC for the best benefit.

Other studies have shown that cannabis users who have IBD have less chance of developing cancer, have fewer hospital days, require fewer surgeries, have fewer infections, and more. That's not to say that cannabis is free of side effects, but if used with a slow introduction and under helpful guidance, it can be a life-changer. People with celiac disease also often turn to cannabis because it helps reduce the symptoms that go along with this condition as well.

Slippery elm and marshmallow root: Both have similar gut-soothing properties because they are rich in mucin, which helps protect the gut by increasing mucus production. Both are also very safe to try and often combined in supplements. These two herbs often work better for people than anti-diarrheal medicines, and they usually deliver the soothing effects that traditional uses promise. Alternatively, you can buy them separately and try them if you wish. It is best to follow the package directions because they come in various forms and doses. See page 308 for recommendations.

Chamomile: Characteristically soothing and rich in anti-inflammatory compounds. For this reason, it has been a gut-healing therapy since the dawn of time. Using chamomile tea is a great option, and you can find chamomile capsules and tinctures as well. The bonus is that it will likely calm your nerves and help you sleep better. See page 305 for recommendations.

Green tea antioxidants: Known as EGCG, helps reduce ulcerative colitis symptoms, even for people who don't respond to conventional treatment,

---

[238] Naftali T, Bar-Lev Schleider L, et al. Cannabis induces a clinical response in patients with Crohn's disease: A prospective placebo-controlled study. *Clin Gastroenterol Hepatol.* 2013 Oct;11(10):1276–80.e1.

according to a small research study.[239] In fact, over half of the people getting the green tea supplement had a 50 percent remission rate compared to zero percent not getting green tea. Both 400 mg and 800 mg doses were effective in this study.

Tulsi (holy basil): You can drink this tea daily, which is well-known to dampen inflammation. It helps counter many kinds of inflammation and stress in the body.

Licorice root: Both soothing and anti-inflammatory, licorice root has been used for ulcerative colitis and Crohn's disease. It is also good for immunity and liver health. Just get DGL licorice to reduce the risk of side effects.

Red Raspberry Leaf: Reduces inflammation and even reduces the risk of cancer—at least, in an animal model of colitis.[240] This type of herb is also safe to use daily and makes a great tea or works in capsule form as well. The other side perk of this herb is that it naturally helps balance hormones.

Turmeric: A review of six clinical trials concluded that turmeric effectively reduces symptoms of ulcerative colitis,[241] which isn't surprising given its anti-inflammatory effects. It is unknown if turmeric works the same way for Crohn's or celiac disease, but it's probably worth a try as long as you aren't sensitive to turmeric. Just make sure to take turmeric with a meal to improve its absorption. It may work even better if you combine it with Boswellia (frankincense).

Other herbs like coriander. Fennel, anise, and peppermint are anti-inflammatory and can be part of a healing diet for IBD. It makes sense to include these herbs in your diet because they help flavor foods. Refer back to Chapter 7 on ways to use these herbs in your daily life.

---

[239] Dryden G, Lam A, et al. A pilot study to evaluate the safety and efficacy of an oral dose of (-)-epigallocatechin-3-gallate-rich polyphenon E in patients with mild to moderate ulcerative colitis. *Inflamm Bowel Dis.* 2013 Aug;19(9):1904–12.

[240] Bibi S, Du M, et al. Dietary red raspberry reduces colorectal inflammation and carcinogenic risk in mice with dextran sulfate sodium-induced colitis. *J Nutr.* 2018 May 1;148(5):667–74.

[241] Zheng T, Wang X, et al. Efficacy of adjuvant curcumin therapy in ulcerative colitis: A meta-analysis of randomized controlled trials. *J Gastroenterol Hepatol.* 2020 May;35(5):722–9.

Case Study: Profound Healing of Ulcerative Colitis with Nourishment

Brent developed ulcerative colitis aged thirty-one. He had been raised on a steady diet of packaged foods and hit the drive through for fast food more often than not for mealtimes. As a child, he had also taken many courses of antibiotics for upper respiratory infections, which wiped out his healthy gut bacteria. Sadly, no one suggested during this time that he take a probiotic supplement. Usually, his gut would respond well to steroid treatments for the colitis, but he was worried about the long term side effects of these medications. In addition to gut symptoms, he struggled with anxiety but couldn't figure out why. He had read a book about how an anti-inflammatory diet could help manage digestive issues like his, and he started following this diet for about a month.

Encouraged by the big improvements in his colitis symptoms, he wanted to add additional healing supplements. After all, he noticed he had fewer flare ups when he added vitamin D3 and cod liver oil, so he wondered if he could also be doing more to protect his gut.

On my advice, he began alternating cooking with bone broth every other day and adding in a grass-fed collagen supplement on the opposite days. Other healthy strategies he adopted were to drink green tea and red raspberry leaf tea daily to also help dampen inflammation. Additionally, he added n-acetylglucosamine once daily, zinc carnosine, is taking organ meats supplements, and added butyrate supplements daily to help heal his gut. To help digest his foods better, he added in raw sauerkraut to support his digestive enzymes and to provide a great source of probiotics. On the days when he couldn't manage to eat sauerkraut, he takes a probiotic with multiple bacillus strains. Last but not least, he added in a low dose cannabis tincture at bedtime to help manage gut pain and to improve his sleep quality.

After another month, he could stop taking the zinc carnosine and skip his probiotic supplements too. He feels like his healing has allowed him to start to cut back on other supplements, too, such as butyrate and cannabis, but he still takes these if he feels colitis symptoms coming on. Overall, he feels

100 percent better than before making these diet and lifestyle changes and has no major colitis flare ups after six months of following this regimen. His anxiety has also diminished, and he rarely feels anxious anymore.

15

Chapter 15

Food Intolerances and Sensitivities: What Helps

A scary thing today is the increasing rates of food intolerance, food sensitivities, and food allergies. Allergic diseases have doubled in less than twenty-five years in industrially-developed countries. Our bodies have become hypersensitive to many things, rooted in immune system issues in the gut and a relative lack of digestive compounds. It is scary because these are signs that your body is on high alert due to inflammation when you have allergies and sensitivities.

Researchers think that food reactions are increasing because of chemicals used in agriculture, food additives like emulsifiers, and overeating processed foods in general. Along with these disturbing trends in food intake comes an increased risk of other gut-related disorders, such as autoimmune diseases. And additives and chemicals continue to increase in our food supply daily.

This means that we all have to be informed consumers of food and put the brakes on eating things that come in packages and that come from factory farms-which is just about everything, sadly. I like to point out that in the 1970s, our food shelves were mostly unprocessed foods and staples.

I remember as a kid going to the grocery store, and there were a few highly processed foods; most were fairly basic canned foods like fruits, vegetables, meats, produce, dairy, and bread. Fast forward to today, where almost every aisle is dominated by heavily processed foods and ingredients—including the freezer and meat sections.

What are Food Intolerances?

Food intolerance is the mildest reaction to foods typically but can be quite uncomfortable nonetheless. It is caused by difficulty digesting a particular food or food eaten after a certain amount. The result is usually discomfort, gas, bloating, or diarrhea/constipation symptoms. If you have a food intolerance, symptoms are only in the gut compared to food sensitivities or allergies. If you react to food in the rest of your body, you likely have a more serious reaction—food sensitivity or food allergy.

I like to point out that you can be intolerant of any food if you eat too much of it because the body's built-in enzyme systems can become overwhelmed if you have a lot of any one thing that your body isn't used to or can't adapt to. Additionally, food chemicals don't digest well and can cause many reactions. As we age, our bodies produce fewer digestive enzymes and stomach acid, which can create new food intolerances that weren't there when we were younger.

The most common food intolerance is lactose. Everyone has their limit with lactose based on their body's ability to make the enzyme called lactase. Lactase helps to break down the lactose sugar in milk. Most people with moderate lactose intolerance can handle eating cheese and yogurt because the probiotic fermentation process of these foods helps to pre-digest the lactose. This is a hint: probiotics can also probably help with lactose intolerance because they build up bacteria that can help you break down lactose.

Other common food intolerances are nightshade vegetables like tomatoes. Also, fructose in fruits like grapes, juices, dried cranberries, sodas, figs, dates, prunes, kiwi, cherries, pears, sweetened yogurt, and apricots. Even a fast-food burger has a high amount of fructose because of all the processed ingredients in the bun! You can also be intolerant of salicylates, which are found in many fruits, vegetables, teas, coffee, spices, nuts, and honey.

Anything that makes you feel off in your gut after eating can indicate intolerance to that food.

Wheat and gluten-containing grains like rye, barley, and some oats are other common food intolerance. Gluten is a protein in grains that is very difficult to digest, and it also comes along with fructans and lectins in grains that can irritate the gut. These **compounds** present difficulties with digestion for many people. Not only can you be intolerant of gluten, but you can also be sensitive and/or allergic, which are signs of more serious immune reactions to these foods.

The most common-sense food advice for dealing with food intolerances is to limit or avoid the foods that cause you issues. An elimination diet in a structured way can be helpful in this case. Additionally, some supplements like probiotics, organ meats, bile acids, betaine HCL, and digestive enzymes can be helpful for some types of food intolerances. We will delve into these more later in this chapter.

Food Sensitivities

Food sensitivities are more serious than food intolerances because your immune system reacts to the food you are eating. This immune reaction can happen in the gut but usually elsewhere in the body. For example, if you commonly have brain fog, achy joints, skin breakouts, etc., you are likely struggling with food sensitivity. Your body recognizes a particular food as a threat, and this causes an inflammatory reaction throughout the body. So, food sensitivities, if left untreated or not managed, can do much damage over time. The increase in food sensitivities these days is thought to be the increasing presence of food additives and chemicals, lack of exposure to healthy bacteria from a young age, and a relative lack of healing foods in most people's so-called "healthy" diets. **Anti-nutrients** present in many foods also can cause sensitivities.

Did You Know . . . It's Difficult to Test for Food Sensitivities

The challenge with identifying food sensitivities is that they can be delayed. You can eat food one day, and your body's immune system can cause its main reaction to it up to four days later. An elimination diet for at least four weeks is a very useful tool. And there aren't any really great lab tests for identifying food sensitivities yet, either. IgG tests can help some people identify food sensitivities. Still, they aren't very accurate because you can have a high IgG level after eating food frequently, even if you aren't sensitive to it. Also, food sensitivity will usually progressively worsen after you eat it for several days in a row.

For example, gluten and wheat-containing products may feel okay when I eat them the first day, but progressively I feel worse if I continue to eat gluten for two to three days in a row. This is a common theme for people with food sensitivities; the more often you eat it, the worse it gets, but its delay makes it challenging to pinpoint. Like food intolerances, food sensitivities can be lessened over time, but they take more serious work on bolstering your immune response with nutrients, healing compounds, and digestive support. In some people, the offending food must be avoided forever.

Food Allergies

The distinction between an allergy and a sensitivity is that a food allergy is usually more immediate in its response; within a few minutes to a couple of hours after eating a certain food, you often will see a reaction, often the skin, lungs, and other systems begin having a relatively strong reaction to a particular food. Food allergies are typically IgE mediated and easier to test for than food sensitivities. The most common food allergies are milk, wheat, soy, egg, peanuts, tree nuts, fish, shellfish, and corn. These foods account for 90 percent of all food allergies.

Because food allergies can become very severe and rapidly worsen, it is best to fully avoid food allergies if you know you have them. While there are some newer food desensitization strategies you can attempt, they must be done under the supervision of someone knowledgeable about food allergies.

Some people do overcome food allergies that they develop as a child, and it is unknown why some people do grow out of them while other people continue to worsen as they get older. Researchers speculate that a leaky gut has much to do with the root causes of food allergies because these reactions are now more common than ever.

If you have food allergies, it's best to avoid them altogether and keep an Epipen nearby for severe allergic reactions like anaphylaxis. But knowing that your gut lining is likely impaired if you have these reactions, you should still focus on healing your gut for the best health- with lots of healthy nutrients, healing compounds, and digestive enzymes as examples of ways to help your whole body in this case.

Advisory: When to Seek Help

Food allergies can be a very serious condition. If you have difficulty breathing, worsening skin reactions or hives, or any other major reaction to foods, you should seek help right away. Generally speaking, it is good to seek help following an elimination diet with a well-trained practitioner such as a functional nutritionist or functional medicine doctor.

Skip the Processed Foods

No question that processed foods accelerates the rates of food sensitivities and allergies. For example, IgE antibodies are four to eight times higher in processed foods than in raw foods in many people, so whenever possible, eat real foods without packages and highly refined foods. It's better to eat a burger on a bed of lettuce and skip the highly processed bun as an example of easy changes to improve your gut's resilience to allergens and toxins.

Be Mindful and Reduce Stress

Stress ramps up allergic responses in the body as well as food sensitivities. This is because stress hormones cause the body to release more histamine. So make sure to keep mealtimes relaxed and comfortable and find ways to manage daily stressors. Many clients have told me that their guts become a wreck when stressed, and an increase in allergic symptoms is a common result.

Many of the herbs and supplements in this book support de-stressing, such as probiotics, chamomile, medicinal mushrooms, and more.

Supplements to Maintain Balance

To calm the immune system down for better food tolerance, it is important to consider adding some supplements to your routine. While food intolerances are milder than food sensitivities or allergies, you may still benefit from many of these to enhance your digestive processes.

Remember that if you have a true food allergy, you should avoid that particular offending food unless under the close supervision of your healthcare provider. And these supplements may lessen symptoms but not necessarily take them away for everyone.

Organ meats: These are perhaps the most important supplement to take if you are trying to heal your gut from food sensitivities, intolerances, and allergies. This is because they contain countless gut-healing compounds the way nature intended them to be. For example, freeze-dried pancreas and gallbladder will give your body natural digestive enzymes and bile to help your body digest your food better. Freeze-dried spleen, thymus, and intestine provide the gut with many immune-balancing compounds that may also heal your gut. And the liver is the most nutrient-dense food on the planet. It does take a leap of faith here because, as I reviewed in previous chapters, we rely on our ancestors who were healers to provide us with this knowledge, as clinical research is lacking in this area. Giving organ meats a try for at least a month is well worth your time, and the risk is extremely low because these foods have been eaten since the dawn of time.

Digestive Enzymes: People who are savvy about gut health almost always have these nearby. They are a godsend for food intolerances and can relieve much of the distress. I even find that some people can tolerate spicy foods or tomatoes when using them. They even can help break down harmful bacteria and yeasts like candida which is good because these harmful microbes can worsen food sensitivities and intolerances. By enhancing the digestibility of proteins in foods, digestive enzymes help dampen down an overactive immune response to foods for people with food sensitivities. Just ensure you get a good broad-spectrum digestive enzyme, as reviewed in Chapter 7, and take them close to the time you eat these foods for the best results.

FODMATE is a specific type of digestive enzyme that helps to digest fermentable carbohydrates, referred to as FODMAPS. This means that people sensitive to things like legumes, vegetables, and fruits may be able to eat moderate amounts of these foods when using this enzyme supplement.

Did You Know . . . Special Enzyme Alert

There is a special enzyme made in the gut that helps break down histamine called diamine oxidase (DAO). Some people don't make enough of this enzyme, which causes allergic symptoms. Additionally, in some people with high histamine levels and who have histamine food triggers, taking DAO supplements can be very helpful.

Bile acids: These are very therapeutic for ongoing diarrhea, but new research even suggests that bile, especially TUDCA, may help our bodies be more tolerant of foods. [242] People with food allergies and sensitivities tend to have lower levels of bile. While more research is needed to prove that bile acids can help food sensitivities, it makes sense to try adding bile supplements if you also have diarrhea and difficulties digesting foods.

---

[242] Virkud Y, Kelly R, et al. The Role of bile acids in food allergy and responses to oral immunotherapy by metabolomic profiling. *The Journal of Allergy and Clinical Immunology.* 2020: 145.

Additionally, if you struggle to tolerate fats in your diet, it may be worth trying to add bile acids to your mealtime, as reviewed in Chapter 7.

Activated Charcoal: This binds to whatever is near, so this can include accidental eating of food allergens or food sensitivities. This is more of a rescue therapy in this sense than a preventive. But, if you know you have a mild sensitivity and occasionally want to enjoy this food, adding a dose of activated charcoal when you eat the food or drink may make your digestive system handle it better, and you will likely have less gas, bloating, and digestive distress.

Ginger: This may reduce food intolerance and food sensitivity reactions because it dampens inflammatory proteins in the gut, all while increasing muscle movements to help prevent indigestion. It is also a natural pain reliever and reduces nausea to boot. Having fresh, pickled, or dried ginger capsules can make you feel better when exposed to offending foods.

Deglycyrrhized (DGL) licorice: Helps regulate immune response by balancing inflammation and T-cells. It also is very healing to intestinal and stomach cells, so it supports a reduction in food allergy and sensitivity for these reasons. Not only that, DGL may reduce cancer risk. Just make sure to find DGL licorice to prevent any unwanted side effects.

Bovine Colostrum: A favorite amongst functional medicine providers for improving immune tolerance because of its ability to gobble up allergen compounds in the gut and its immune-balancing effects. This is my go-to for many kinds of sensitivities, including seasonal allergies. Just avoid bovine colostrum if you have a true milk allergy.

Chlorella: Gut-related problems, including food sensitivities, can be rooted in toxic exposures. The major action of chlorella is to bind and remove toxins like heavy metals from the gut. It also reduces the release of histamine from cells, so it can dampen histamine food sensitivity.

Quercetin with Vitamin C: These natural antioxidants have a double duty of reducing histamine levels in the body, so they can be great for temporarily relieving mild food allergies, food sensitivities, or reactions to histamine foods. Be aware that quercetin can slow down your caffeine metabolism, which means your morning coffee may be extra potent if you take quercetin.

Apple cider vinegar with the mother: While a useful indigestion remedy, apple cider vinegar can be part of a holistic routine for reducing food sensitivities and intolerances for some. By naturally helping balance the pH in your body and providing natural probiotics, it stands to reason it may help. It's mostly a folk remedy, but research does show that it reduces inflammation and blood pressure, so it's definitely not inactive in the body.[243] You can try apple cider vinegar (with the mother) capsules to see if it helps your tolerance of offending foods.

Probiotics and Prebiotics: We have become too hygienic in some ways as a society, which is likely at the root of the increase in food allergies and sensitivities. Probiotics help to improve immune tolerance and calm down overreactions to our foods and the world around us. For example, in children with cow's milk sensitivity, Bifidobacterium probiotics reduce the severity of skin rashes due to cow's milk. It also reduces the symptoms of seasonal allergies in adults. Probiotics are probably most successful in reducing food sensitivities and allergies if given to people early in life, even before birth and during infancy.

And here is the irony: people who have healthier guts have a better response to probiotics than those who don't have healthy guts. This shouldn't be a deterrent from probiotics if your gut isn't healthy, but an endorsement for bolstering your gut health with many strategies and adding probiotics.

Prebiotics can help support the use of probiotics by helping to keep these probiotics thriving in the gut-but much less work has been done to determine the degree of effectiveness of prebiotics for people with allergies and sensitivities.

Vitamins and minerals: If you are low in any nutrient, it can compromise the health and strength of the gut lining. When the gut lining is inflamed and compromised, the body is more likely to react to the foods you eat negatively. It is extra important to take vitamins and minerals if you don't eat organ

---

[243] Gheflati A, Bashiri R, et al. The effect of apple vinegar consumption on glycemic indices, blood pressure, oxidative stress, and homocysteine in patients with type 2 diabetes and dyslipidemia: A randomized controlled clinical trial. *Clin Nutr ESPEN.* 2019 Oct;33:132–8.

meats. Adding extra vitamin A as vitamin A palmitate and vitamin D3 will likely be beneficial, too, because of the healing properties they can provide the gut by helping prevent allergens from entering the body.

Immunoglobulins-IgG immunoglobulins are similar to colostrum because they help to gobble up allergens in the gut and is more suitable for people who have milk allergy than colostrum. Often people find that they can tolerate foods they previously couldn't tolerate after using IgG supplements for about a month, although clinical trials are needed to prove this benefit.

Butyrate-Is healing for the gut and may reduce food sensitivity reactions by balancing immune cells. Many people find it is overall balancing for digestion and it is even good for liver health. Typical doses are 1-2 grams twice daily, but you can start with around 500 mg twice daily to see how it works for you.

Medicinal Mushrooms can help support a balanced immunity which may help improve food tolerance over time. Popular mushrooms for use to prevent allergy symptoms are Reishi mushrooms and Lion's mane mushrooms. You can get a mushroom powder and add it to your favorite drink but don't expect it to be a quick fix.

Green tea may dampen the allergic response to food allergies because it dampens histamine release in the body if used regularly. An easy way to incorporate green tea into the diet is to swap it out for coffee or other beverages.

Tryptophan is an amino acid that helps make serotonin, the happy mood chemical. Early research also shows that tryptophan in the form of 5-hydroxytryptophan (5-HTP) may reduce food allergic responses too. Make sure to take tryptophan with plenty of B vitamins, especially niacin, for its full benefit. I personally like to combine it with tyrosine as reviewed in the Postbiotics section of Chapter 8.

Case Study: Finding Enjoyment in Mealtimes Again

Cindy seemed to have more food sensitivities and intolerances the older she got. While her symptoms were manageable, everything she ate caused flatulence. She also was sure that her skin rashes and breakouts were due to food sensitivities too. In the spring and summer, her seasonal allergies would rage, but she would limp along with the use of antihistamines. Her doctor ruled out the possibility of IBS, so it was determined that she was likely sensitive to foods.

At first, Cindy tried to eliminate the main food culprits, including some dairy products, wheat, and beans. This helped but didn't fix the problem. So she embarked on a full elimination diet, which mostly fixed the issues, but she would still struggle a few days of the week with bloating. She also started drinking green tea daily and adding medicinal mushroom powder to her foods daily. Luckily her skin mostly cleared in about six weeks, so she knew she was on the right track.

Fast forward two years. Cindy really missed some of her favorite foods like beans, tomatoes, dairy, and bread, so she sought out my help to determine if there was anything else she could do. The first and most important change she agreed to make was to add a broad-spectrum digestive enzyme along with a FODMATE digestive supplement and bile acids called TUDCA to any meal that she suspected would cause her distress. She also started taking her natural vitamins and minerals more consistently and added a teaspoon of colostrum powder twice daily. She also agreed to take butyrate daily.

After doing so, eating fermented beans, dairy, and fresh tomatoes was not a problem now if she only ate them in moderation. Sadly she still couldn't tolerate much wheat, but she could sneak a slice of pizza occasionally without any major digestive problems. But happy to be rid of most of her sensitivities, she can now enjoy most of the foods she thought she would have to avoid forever. For her seasonal allergies, she added in 1 g of liposomal vitamin C daily, nettles, and a quercetin supplement during the spring and summer, and now she could even skip taking her over-the-counter antihistamines. Using the colostrum was very helpful in reducing her seasonal allergies too. By doing so, she had much more energy because she didn't need the antihistamine supplements anymore and could enjoy spring and summer the way she always wanted to.

16

Chapter 16

Gallbladder Issues: Diet and Supplement Strategies

Almost a million gallbladders are removed annually in the United States alone, with at least 10-15 percent of the population suffering from gallbladder disease. It seems unimaginable, but over 5 billion dollars are spent on gallbladder surgery yearly, and the trend isn't improving. These organs are removed, then the resulting imbalances can create lifelong digestive struggles with eating after the surgery too. And women are much more likely than men to get gallstones related to hormone issues.

Sadly, gallbladder disease is mostly preventable and even treatable using natural approaches if caught early. That's not to say that gallbladder surgery isn't necessary because it can be a necessary and life-saving procedure. But at the root of most gallbladder issues are inflammation and imbalances from food, so diet and nutrient intake can dramatically change your risk. And gallbladder removal increases the risk of a host of other diseases like metabolic syndrome diseases, so it shouldn't be taken lightly. These diseases include fatty liver disease, diabetes, weight gain, and increased blood cholesterol. Prevention is a better strategy than removal of the gallbladder when possible.

Did You Know . . . Amazing Gallbladder Facts

The gallbladder's microbiome reflects the microbiome of your mouth. Harmful bacteria from the top down create an altered microbiome that promotes gallstone formation. Another fact that supports how important the microbiome is: probiotics are effective at helping prevent gallstones for people who have previously had a gallstone-promoting surgery called bariatric surgery.

The understanding that the microbiome has played a role in the health of the gallbladder isn't new. As far back as the early 1900s, a medical textbook by William Osler noted that toxins in the blood cause damage to liver function, which directly affects the health of the gallbladder. These toxins, we now know, are harmful microbes that enter the bloodstream from the gut.

Healing the gut with diet and nutritional strategies should be the goal for preventing and managing gallbladder conditions. By doing so, you can help prevent harmful microbes from entering the gallbladder and the liver.

Gallbladder Basics

The gallbladder, looking at it most simplistically, is the storage vessel for bile. Bile helps the body absorb and emulsify fats from your diet. The bile is made in the liver and then descends into the gallbladder for storage. The gallbladder is part of a branching network of digestive support called the biliary tree. Below the gallbladder within the biliary tree are the bile duct and the pancreatic duct, where pancreatic enzymes are released.

It's all connected. So as you can imagine, if you have inflammation in the gallbladder or your liver, the odds are that you are also inflamed in the area where the pancreas releases its enzymes. This means that if you suffer from a gallbladder issue, you most likely are not getting enough pancreatic enzymes, and your liver is probably not at its best, either.

Gallbladder Disorders

The gallbladder can have more issues than gallstones, but they all tie back to imbalances related to diet, microbiome, and inflammation. Here are the most common gallbladder conditions.

- Gallstones are "stones" made up of crystallized bile that form because of poor bile flow, inadequate bile salts, or a buildup of cholesterol in the bile. Up to 80 percent of people with gallstones never have an issue, yet gallstones are the leading cause of GI-related hospitalizations. Most gallstones are benign, but 20 percent cause major issues.
- Cholecystitis is inflammation in the gallbladder related to poor flow of bile and can be caused by gallstones and poor diet and nutrition habits.
- Cholangitis is an infection in the biliary tree due to a blockage of bile flow, and it can be very dangerous because it can lead to a liver infection. This condition needs immediate medical attention.
- Gallstone pancreatitis is where a gallstone blocks the pancreas and is also very dangerous and needs urgent attention.

Did You Know . . . When to Seek Help

Some signs of gallstone issues are sudden pain on the right side of your belly or right shoulder. People suffering from gallstones also can have nausea and vomiting out of the blue. If you have gallstones and you have pain that won't go away after an hour or two, or you have a fever, you should make sure to see a doctor. Or, if you have ongoing weight loss and poor appetite, you should also see your doctor.

How Diet Helps or Hurts

If your diet is not balanced due to processed foods, the gallbladder suffers no matter who you are. These processed foods lead to an altered microbiome and imbalances in the liver and contribute to a leaky gut which allows unwanted bacteria and germs to enter your bloodstream. This situation creates inflammation in the liver which then results in slow bile flow. But for most people, the problem is fixable and preventable.

Processed foods to steer clear of to help avoid gallbladder issues are sugar, sodas, chips, other fried foods, most crackers, baked goods, trans fats, and processed seed oils like vegetable oil and canola oil. These foods also cause estrogen imbalances which contribute to gallstones. Additionally, heavy metals are often present in high amounts in gallstones, so eating a diet that helps to clear heavy metals from the body also makes sense. Interestingly, antibiotics increase the uptake of heavy metals in the body, so you should only use antibiotic medications when necessary.

In contrast, if you eat a diet full of healthy nutrients and probiotics, the opposite happens. The liver becomes more balanced, inflammation decreases, and the microbiome becomes restored. And a healthy diet includes lots of fresh vegetables, herbs, spices, proteins, healthy fats like extra virgin olive oil, fermented vegetables, and more. A great meal plan for gallbladder health is a Paleo-style diet where processed sugars, fats, and grains are eliminated or minimized.

Foods that can help safely remove heavy metals from the body and promote gallbladder health include cilantro and broken cell wall chlorella. Pectin-rich foods like apples, oranges, other citrus, sweet potatoes, green beans, and plums also help to bind and remove unwanted heavy metals. The citrus pith or white part that holds the fruit together is especially high in pectin. Probiotic foods like sauerkraut, kimchi, and yogurt also help to restore gut health and even can help bind heavy metals and remove them from the body. Just make sure that your yogurt is unsweetened for the best health.

For estrogen balance, it is good to include broccoli sprouts, raw broccoli, arugula, brussels sprouts, organ meats, and all the other healthy foods discussed above.

Contrary to popular belief, weight loss only contributes to gallstones if eaten on a low-fat (high-carb) diet. Weight loss related to a low-carb, higher-fat diet does not increase the risk of gallstones, according to a review of thirteen clinical trials. [244] This all points to processed carbs as the biggest culprits for gallbladder disease, not fat.

And last but not least, gluten may also cause gallbladder disease. Gallbladder disease is much more common among people with celiac disease and gluten sensitivity-whether people know it or not-before gallbladder issues occur. Other food sensitivities also likely increase the risk of gallbladder disease because they cause inflammation and cause the body to mount an immune response. If you suspect you have gluten sensitivity, you should try to minimize or avoid gluten, and if you have celiac disease, you should avoid gluten entirely. You can refer to Chapter 15 for more help with food sensitivities.

Targeted Foods to Eat for Gallbladder Health

Gallbladder issues often result in nausea and discomfort after meals or at random times. This nausea is a trigger that something needs to change, including your diet. Nausea can be due to poor absorption of foods due to gallbladder inflammation, gallstones, and more. If you have severe pain or gallbladder issues, seek emergency help. But, if your symptoms are mild or you just want to keep your gallbladder and biliary tree healthy, here are some foods you should focus on eating.

Celery juice: Celery is rich in medicinal compounds that are healthy for the gallbladder, liver, and digestive tract. It helps neutralize all sorts of toxins, so it would make sense that it can help the gallbladder too. While you can eat celery, too, celery juice is a very concentrated way to get more celery in your diet.

Apple cider vinegar: A long-time folk remedy for gallstone issues, apple cider vinegar certainly is worth a try. Just make sure to dilute it either with water or use it in recipes because it is very strong. The best kinds of apple

---

[244] Stokes C, Gluud L, et al. Ursodeoxycholic acid and diets higher in fat prevent gallbladder stones during weight loss: A meta-analysis of randomized controlled trials. *Clin Gastroenterol Hepatol.* 2014 Jul;12(7):1090–1100.e2; quiz e6.

cider vinegar are the ones that contain the mother.

Extra virgin olive oil: This is both protective for liver and gallbladder health due to its high polyphenol content, so it is a smart kind of fat to include with every meal, especially if you have gallbladder issues. In the Mediterranean, people eat around 9 tablespoons of olive oil daily and have very healthy gallbladders. Eating at least 2 tablespoons a day reduces gallstone risk. Don't substitute refined olive oil.

Apples: The malic acid in apples helps to soften gallstones.

Bitters: Bitter foods like arugula, celery, broccoli, endive, dandelion, burdock root, and Brussels sprouts help stimulate bile flow from the gallbladder. Herbal bitter supplements can also be used, and many people find they are very effective in helping digestive issues like gallbladder disease.

Taurine-rich foods: Help make bile salts, so it is important to have taurine in the diet. These foods include grass-fed meats, wild-caught fish, and algae. Anxiety, autism, hypertension, gout, infertility, and obesity may be conditions of low taurine levels.

Herbs and spices: The more variety, the better. For example, turmeric helps the gallbladder empty so that stones are less likely to form. Ginger likely increases bile flow too. Garlic may help dissolve gallstones, while coriander and other herbs and spices dampen gallbladder inflammation.

Supplements for Gallbladder Health

You can't have a healthy gallbladder if your gut is leaky and the gut lining is inflamed. An imbalance in bacteria also creates a broken gut and negatively affects the gallbladder. For these reasons, supplements that are healing for the gut are also protective of the gallbladder.

Here are some other supplement options for improving bile flow. Generally, you should follow the package directions for supplementation and, as always, check with a healthcare provider well-versed in natural health before starting anything new.

Probiotics: An altered microbiome, starting in the mouth, is one of the causal factors behind gallbladder disease. Gallbladder removal further disrupts the microbiome, increasing the risk of abdominal cancers, sadly. Probiotics can reduce the incidence of gallbladder disease and promote a healthy balance of bile, helps reduce cholesterol, and reduces inflammation. Therefore, it makes sense to include healthy probiotics in the diet from fermented foods, and so does taking a probiotic supplement if you are suffering from gallbladder issues or want to help prevent them. A broad-spectrum probiotic with *Lactobacillus* and *Bifidobacterium* is your best bet, but you can also try *Bacillus* strains for ease of tolerance.

Prebiotics: Especially acacia, pectin, and other gentle fibers may be soothing and beneficial for gallbladder disease because it stimulates butyrate production and probiotics. Fiber also helps to prevent gallbladder sludge formation.

Ox bile: When your gallbladder isn't working well, your body isn't getting enough bile to digest and absorb the fats you eat. This can cause further inflammation, nausea, and pain. Adding ox bile can at least help alleviate some nausea related to gallbladder issues or for people who have had their gallbladder removed. It also can help heal the gut by promoting nutrient absorption. Some people choose to supplement grass-fed beef gallbladder instead. You can also use TUDCA, which is essentially bile salts with taurine. Research shows that using a combination of TUDCA and probiotics reduces gallstone formation.[245]

Digestive enzymes: If your gallbladder isn't working well or you just had your gallbladder removed, digestive enzymes can alleviate a lot of nausea and pain for many people. They also dampen inflammation, which is a win-win for the gallbladder and the gut. Just make sure to take them each time you eat food. Review the best digestive enzymes in Chapter 8.

Vitamins and minerals: Nutrients that dampen inflammation are critical for gallbladder health, including vitamin D, vitamin A, and selenium. Taking organ meats and/or a broad-spectrum multivitamin with minerals is a smart

---

[245] Gao F, Guan D, et al. Effects of oral tauroursodeoxycholic acid and/or intestinal probiotics on serum biochemical indexes and bile composition in patients with cholecystolithiasis. *Front Pharmacol*. 2022 Oct 24;13:882764.

idea for everyone, including people who want to prevent gallbladder issues.

Magnesium: This helps promote liver function and is necessary for gut and gallbladder health. Most people are deficient in magnesium, so it makes sense to supplement with magnesium and get adequate magnesium in the diet by eating more leafy greens, dark chocolate, and pumpkin seeds. Magnesium malate is a good choice, as is magnesium taurate or magnesium glycinate. Use a moderate dose as the label recommends, or you can get an unwanted laxative effect. It also makes sense to regularly take Epsom salt baths which are magnesium sulfate-based.

Cod liver oil: This is important, especially if you don't regularly eat fish. Its anti-inflammatory effects and benefits to blood fats are indispensable for all-around health, including the gallbladder and gut. This highly absorbable form of omega-3 fats also provides natural vitamin A. See page 305 for recommendations.

Supplements that Promote Bile Flow

Mild gallbladder issues can be helped with diet and supplement tips like the following. Keep in mind that our bodies aren't reductionist like research is. This means using multiple natural approaches and remedies at a time is often your best bet.

Did You Know . . . You Can Promote Gallbladder with a Supplement Regime.

Research shows a multi-pronged approach helps promote gallbladder function best. For example, one clinical study found that a supplement called A-F Betafood by Standard Process that contains beet leaf, carrot powder, beet powder, magnesium citrate, bovine liver, bovine prostate, yeast, vitamin A palmitate, bovine kidney, alfalfa, flaxseed, orchic extract, vitamin C, iodine, lecithin, and vitamin E helped to improve gallbladder function in people with gallbladder insufficiency.[246] [247]This supplement is available on Fullscript.

So trying several of these remedies simultaneously, along with the ones above, makes the most sense. For example, you could use digestive enzymes, ox bile, lemon, organ meats, apple cider vinegar, magnesium, stone breaker, probiotics, and bitters to have a synergistic effect. Depending on your baseline diet, you might benefit from a slightly different regimen, such as probiotics, milk thistle, turmeric, cardamom, TUDCA, cod liver oil, and malic acid.

Milk thistle: Helps protect the liver and biliary tree because it is rich in antioxidants, supports healthy immunity, and balances. It also is thought to help stimulate bile flow and is a safe herb to take unless you are allergic to it.

Bitters: These are useful supplements to take to promote bile flow. You can find bitters both in tincture and capsule form, and they are usually a blend of edible anti-inflammatory herbs.

Mullein: A very helpful herb for many digestive concerns, including gallbladder issues.

Cardamom: A traditional treatment for just about every digestive ailment, including gallbladder sludge, gallstones, and inflammation.

Turmeric. This helps the gallbladder empty. You can supplement turmeric if you don't like this spice in your diet.

Beetroot: Helps the gallbladder in numerous ways by dampening inflammation and improving cholesterol levels. It also helps clear out toxins like heavy metals from the body too.

Supplements That Reduce Gallstones

The following supplements benefit people trying to prevent or treat mild gallstone disease. Keep in mind that these supplements can't replace a

---

[246]Tint G, Salen G, et al Ursodeoxycholic acid: A safe and effective agent for dissolving cholesterol gallstones. *Ann Intern Med.* 1982 Sep;97(3):351–6.

[247]Evans M, Guthrie N, et al. A whole-food-based health product (A-F Betafood®) improves gallbladder function in humans at risk of gallbladder insufficiency: A randomized, placebo-controlled clinical trial. *Nutrients.* 2020 Feb 20;12(2):540.

healthy diet, as discussed above, and that you still should always seek help from a knowledgeable healthcare provider for your own unique needs before adding any of these to your regimen.

Stone breaker herb: Aptly named because it helps reduce stone formation in the body. This is because it helps alkalize the body. So stone breaker herb may also help reduce existing gallstones and improve bile flow. While research is lacking, countless individuals swear it has made a tremendous difference in their gallbladder health. It also helps reduce kidney stones too.

TUDCA: As mentioned before is very helpful when combined with probiotics to reduce gallstones. It is best when taken with meals, and it also has a host of other health benefits for reducing inflammation and promoting heart health.

Garlic Oil: Helps soften gallstones, according to early research.[248] Since garlic is a safe herb for everyone, it's worth a try when added to a healthy diet and supplements. You can even find garlic oil combined with mullein in a supplement; see page 306 for recommendations.

Taurine: An amino acid that is part of TUDCA supplements. Still, it also may help alone for gallbladders, especially for people with low taurine diets, such as vegetarians and vegans. Taurine helps reduce cholesterol buildup in the gallbladder, according to early research. [249]

Lemon: The antioxidants in lemons and the peel are thought to help soften gallstones, and some research indicates that it may help with this condition.[250]

Malic acid: This is present in apples and is thought to be the compound responsible for helping soften gallstones. It is naturally anti-inflammatory as well and even helps reduce fibromyalgia pain.

Vitamin C: Consistently is linked with fewer gallstones because it may help

---

[248] Nijhawan S, Agarwal V, et al. Evaluation of garlic oil as a contact dissolution agent for gallstones: comparison with monooctanoin. *Trop Gastroenterol.* 2000 Oct–Dec;21(4):177–9.

[249] Yamanaka Y, Tsuji K, et al. Effect of dietary taurine on cholesterol gallstone formation and tissue cholesterol contents in mice. *J Nutr Sci Vitaminol (Tokyo).* 1985 Apr;31(2):225–32.

[250] Igimi H, Hisatsugu T, et al. The use of d-limonene preparation as a dissolving agent of gallstones. *Am J Dig Dis.* 1976 Nov;21(11):926–39.

soften and reduce stones, according to research.[251] Studies use 500 mg a day, given several times a day for this purpose.

Peppermint oil: Supports a healthy gallbladder by reducing inflammation, relaxing the gallbladder, and reducing nausea related to gallbladder inflammation. It may work even better when combined with caraway oil, according to research.[252]

Organ Meats: These contain hundreds of healing compounds and nutrients, such as phosphatidylcholine, that help reduce stone-forming tendencies.

Phosphatidylcholine: This makes cholesterol in the gallbladder more dissolvable.

N-acetylcysteine: helps dissolve gallstones in very preliminary research.[253] It does so by acting to reduce mucin, which is part of gallstone formation. This supplement is also an antioxidant that helps health generally.

Hormone Balance Supplements

Imbalance in estrogen levels, both for men and women, can cause a lot of health issues and contributes to gallbladder issues as well. Several foods and supplements help improve estrogen balance.

Cruciferous vegetables, especially eaten raw, help to detoxify estrogen, so they may help reduce gallbladder issues as well. These vegetables include broccoli sprouts, broccoli, arugula, Brussels sprouts, radishes, etc. While you can work on adding more of these to your diet, some people simply can't tolerate these bitter foods when eaten raw.

---

[251] Simon J, Hudes E. Serum ascorbic acid and other correlates of gallbladder disease among US adults. *Am J Public Health.* 1998 Aug;88(8):1208–12.

[252] Goerg K, Spilker T. Effect of peppermint oil and caraway oil on gastrointestinal motility in healthy volunteers: a pharmacodynamic study using simultaneous determination of gastric and gall-bladder emptying and orocaecal transit time. *Aliment Pharmacol Ther.* 2003 Feb;17(3):445–51.

[253] Niu N, Smith BF. Addition of N-acetylcysteine to aqueous model bile systems accelerates dissolution of cholesterol gallstones. Gastroenterology. 1990 Feb;98(2):454–63.

Here is a partial list of helpful supplements for estrogen imbalances.

Broccoli sprouts extract: Particularly helpful for balancing hormones because they are up to 100 times more potent than broccoli florets.

Red raspberry leaf: An all-around health tonic that is thought to help support the integrity of the gallbladder by helping to balance hormones in the body. This herb is especially helpful for people with estrogen dominance. It is found almost anywhere as a tea, or you can supplement this helpful herb.

Chaste berry: Known as a women's tonic herb, chaste berry (vitex) has many possible benefits. It is especially useful at low doses, where it helps to reduce estrogen dominance and supports overall hormonal health. It helps to reduce constipation and helps improve mood too. Check with your functional medicine provider if you are trying to get pregnant, have PCOS, or are currently pregnant.

A herbal blend can help balance estrogen dominance and low progesterone levels. Again, double-check with your healthcare provider, but taking an herbal blend called Women's Phase I by Vitanica changed my life for the better in many ways. See page 309 for recommendations.

Case Study: Kicking Gallstones to the Curb

Mark's digestion was definitely off because he would get pain and nausea when eating fried chicken wings, pizza, or any fast food. His doctor determined that he had moderate gallbladder disease that could be watched and didn't require surgery immediately.

By cleaning up his diet, he was able to reduce many of the symptoms but sought out advice to see if there could be a way to help manage his gallbladder symptoms naturally. After changing his diet to mostly unprocessed foods, destressing his life, and focusing on having a lot of anti-inflammatory foods like fish, extra virgin olive oil, fruits, and vegetables, he felt better most of the time. He also avoided gluten and avoided convenience foods and took a daily probiotic. All of these things helped a lot, but he still had some gallbladder symptoms remaining.

We explored additional nutritional approaches, and he agreed to try the following:

- Stone breaker herb tincture one dropper twice daily.
- Celery juice with bitter herbs 1 cup daily.
- Liposomal vitamin C 500 mg three times daily.
- Betafood® 2 tablets with each meal.
- Cod liver oil 2 gelcaps.
- Lemon water several times a day.
- Extra dietary garlic.
- Magnesium 150 mg per day.
- Mullein tea daily.

After just a week of this routine, Mark's symptoms were virtually gone. I encouraged him to continue this remedy for another week and then periodically to support his gallbladder health. He no longer struggles with gallbladder issues and could go off of everything but his extra magnesium, cod liver oil, vitamin C, and Betafood. He still gets regular follow up with his doctor and eats junk food only occasionally, but there is no indication of the need for surgery.

17

Chapter 17

Conclusion

Happy Gut Healing Ever After

Digestive conditions are the costliest conditions in our world today, yet simple healing strategies can help many people feel so much better. At the root of most digestive issues is a lack of healing nutrients and compounds. Luckily, you don't have to live in a gut-depleted world because you can use several diet strategies and supplements to help heal your gut given throughout this book.

I hope that the information provided in this book has given you hope for healing and some simple steps to improve your gut health and overall health. It is important to note that we are all unique, so you may find yourself exploring various healing options. You may also find that trying a more intensive healing process, meaning more than one supplement and diet strategy at once, may help you heal faster and get the maximum improvement in your gut health.

Turning toward ancestral healing backed by modern science is truly the cutting edge of gut health. But the learning doesn't stop here. I encourage each and every one of you to be curious about your own health, use the

National Library of Medicine, and become savvy at discovering your own best path. Be your own health advocate, be curious, and ask questions about your gut health. If you aren't getting any solutions to your gut issues with conventional approaches, I encourage you to use this book as a reference and seek out a functional medicine provider that can address your own unique needs.

I can't emphasize enough that knowledge is power, and learning should continue constantly. Each day, new research is released that advocates for using natural medicines. So find a research study, give it to your doctor, and discuss it.

As always, use a risk versus benefit approach-many of these supplements hold little risk, but if you are allergic to or sensitive to anything, you should always honor that and avoid it.

You should also share this book with your loved ones because they will then better understand why you are taking the path you are taking. As a benefit, they may also find ways to help their own health.

18

Chapter 18

Recommended Supplements

In order to ensure that you get a high-quality supplement, it is best to purchase the following brands directly from the companies listed below or through Fullscript, which is a dispensary where supplements are approved by health professionals and quality is guaranteed.

To buy from Fullscript, you will need to have your own healthcare professional provide you with an account. Alternatively, you can use my account at https://us.fullscript.com/welcome/hmoretti/. Disclosure: I make a small affiliate income if you use this link.

A-F Betafood: is a healthy blend of vegetables, herbs, and organ meats designed to support a healthy gallbladder and digestive tract. Available on Fullscript.

Apple Cider Vinegar: You can find a good apple cider vinegar supplement from Enzymedica or Now Foods on Fullscript.

Bile Salts: A pharmaceutical-grade ox bile supplement is Seeking Health Ox Bile from the Seeking Health website or Body Bio TUDCA, available on Fullscript.

Butyrate: You can find a high-quality butyrate supplement from a company called Body Bio.

Caraway and Peppermint: IB Care or Caraway: Dyspepsia Complex by Terravita from Canada contains both mint and caraway at a dose of 450 mg, which is not in the oil form. Hence, its dosing is different from the oil mentioned in the studies.

Chamomile: Medi Herb and Herb Pharm are good brands of chamomile that you can find on Fullscript or directly from the company.

Chlorella: Some good chlorella brands are Chlorella Plus from Douglas Laboratories and Now Organic Chlorella. Both are available on Fullscript and in retail health food stores or dispensaries.

Cod liver oil: Get high-quality brands such as Standard Process or Vital Nutrients.

Collagen: Grassfed Living Collagen, Amy Myers, MD, and Wholesome Wellness are a few reputable brands that contain all three types of collagen. You can find these on Amazon and in some natural health food stores.

Colostrom; The colostrum that I recommend and use is Sovereign Laboratories Colostrum LD because they use liposomal colostrum. You can buy it directly from the company online and you can use my affiliate link here: https://shareasale.com/r.cfm?b=402166&u=2131528&m=42760&urllink=&afftrack=.

Digestive Enzymes: I recommend Pure Encapsulations, Seeking Health, Amy Myers, MD, Integrative Therapeutics, Designs for Health, and Klaire Labs.

Electrolytes: A good electrolyte drink that I use is Seeking Health Optimal Electrolyte Powder. You can also get electrolytes in tablet form at Fullscript.

Garlic (as stabilized allicin): Allimax is a reputable brand of stabilized allicin, and you can find it on Fullscript or direct from the company. Another good option is Allicidin by Premier Research Laboratories.

Garlic Oil: You can find garlic oil combined with mullein in a supplement in the Seeking Health brand or Dr. Amy Myers brand.

Ginger and Peppermint: Heather's Tummy Tamers are available directly from their website, or you can also find them on Amazon. Because they sell directly from the company on Amazon, it is a safe product to purchase here.

The only difference between this product and the kind used in research is that Heather's Tummy Tamers also contains fennel, which is good for gut health too.

Glutamine: Dr. Amy Myers Gut Repair or Pure Encapsulations L-Glutamine Powder are good brand options. Another option is Leaky Gut Revive by Amy Myers, MD, and you can find it on her website.

IgG (Immunoglobulin G): A reputable brand is Microbiome Labs which is available on Fullscript or directly from the company.

Lavender: A pharmaceutical-grade lavender oil gel cap brand on the market is highly rated. It is called Lavella by Integrative Therapeutics, which you can find in some health food stores or on Fullscript.

Magnesium: Calm brand of magnesium is available on Fullscript and also in most major retailers.

Medicinal Mushrooms: My favorite brands are Medicinal Foods, Fresh Cap, and Real Mushrooms. These brands are all USDA organic and third-party certified.

MegaGuard: contains artichoke leaf extract, GutGard licorice extract (DGL), and ginger root. This combination is great to alleviate many digestive symptoms like heartburn, gas, indigestion, and more. Available on Fullscript.

Milk Thistle: Reputable supplement and brands include Designs for Health and Jarrow.

Mullein: Available from Fullscript, a good mullein supplement is Gaia Mighty Lungs.

Omega-3 Fats: Standard Process and Vital Nutrients through Fullscript.

Oregano: Candibactin-AR and Intestinol by Orthomolecular herbal therapy for SIBO, available on Fullscript.

Organ Meats: The brands I consistently use for organ meats are MK Supplements and Ancestral Supplements. Both brands carry unique organ meat supplements—both are sourced from 100 percent grass-fed cattle. These companies freeze-dry the organ meats so all the digestive factors and enzymes remain intact. I encourage you to go to their website, browse the reviews for these products and decide for yourself. You can find MK Supplements at * https://shop.michaelkummer.com?aff=10 and you can find

Ancestral Supplements directly from their website. *affiliate link

Peppermint: For adults, a good peppermint supplement is called Peppermint Oil GI, which also contains ginger and fennel. It is meant to be used periodically if you struggle with many GI symptoms.

Probiotics: Some brands of probiotics that are high quality are Megaspore Biotic and Florastor. Microbiome Labs MegasporeBiotic has the most research behind it, and it is my preferred probiotic for myself and my family. Or, for a gentle formula, try Probiotic Restoraflora by Microbiome Labs. These are available on Fullscript.

Quercetin: You can find pharmaceutical-grade quercetin from Pure Encapsulations or Jarrow Formulas at many retail health food stores or on Fullscript.

Slippery elm and marshmallow root: Vital Nutrients and Dr. Amy Myers both have GI repair powders that contain both ingredients.

Thyme: Although somewhat more difficult to find, you can usually get a thyme tincture from herbal stores or from a company online called Herb Pharm.

Turmeric: Available in most retail pharmacies, but Gaia and Klaire Labs are reputable brands. Just make sure to take turmeric with food.

Vitamins and Minerals: You will usually find the following natural brands in health food stores and online from companies like Fullscript (or directly from the company):

- Amy Myers MD
- Designs for Health
- Garden of Life Vitamin Code
- Integrative Therapeutics
- Klaire Laboratories
- Pure Encapsulations
- Seeking Health
- Solgar
- Thorne

Thyme: Candibactin-AR and Intestinol by Orthomolecular herbal therapy for SIBO, available in health food stores or on Fullscript.

Tulsi: Organic India, available in health food stores or on Fullscript.

Turmeric: I like Gaia's professional-grade turmeric found in health food stores or on Fullscript. Also, Douglas Labs carries a Boswellia-turmeric complex with the additive anti-inflammatory benefit of Boswellia in it.

Zinc carnosine: For zinc carnosine, good brands include Pure Encapsulations or Integrative Therapeutics through Fullscript.

Other Remedies

Motion sickness: Sinus Plumber is a homeopathic sinus spray that helps alleviate sinus congestion and pressure. Available in some health food stores and on Amazon. It contains some horseradish and capsaicin, so it initially has a burning sensation followed by relief. For a more mild feeling, you can try Sinu Orega-also available on Amazon.

Pain relief: Try cannabis salve, Icy Hot, capsaicin patches or cream, diluted topical essential oils, BioFreeze, etc.

Hormone balance: Women's Phase I by Vitanica produced by Vitanica, is a blend of herbs designed to help reduce hormonal symptoms, and I love it for helping regulate menstrual cycles. It contains natural borage, wild yam, dandelion root, dong quai, and chaste tree. You can find this in local herbal stores or on Amazon.

19

Chapter 19

Glossary

Adhesions: scar tissue that forms from surgical procedures that causes two types of tissues to be connected that should not be connected.

Antinutrients: A natural or synthetic compound that blocks the absorption of nutrients.

Antinutritional: Compounds that block the absorption of nutrients and absorption of other healthy compounds.

Antioxidants: Dietary compounds are generally considered healthy because they reduce free radicals in the body by dampening the oxidation process.

Ayurvedic medicine: An ancient medical system that continues to be used alongside conventional medicine in India today. This type of medicine includes diet, herbs, exercise, and lifestyle.

Compounds: Any substance made from two or more bonded elements.

Cortisol: A hormone made by your adrenal glands that are made in response to stress, but it is also a necessary hormone that balances metabolism and immunity.

Desiccation: Use of chemicals to interrupt plant growth after seed size has been set.

Digestive diseases: Disorders of the digestive tract or gastrointestinal tract.

Fight-or-flight response: A physical reaction to an event that the body senses as stressful or frightening.

Free-radical: Unstable particles that can damage cells and contribute to many illnesses and aging.

GERD: An acronym for gastroesophageal reflux disease caused by stomach contents flowing into the esophagus.

H. pylori: A type of bacteria that can infect the stomach and cause a host of digestive issues.

Inflammation: When tissue becomes hot, red, swollen, or painful. It happens when the body triggers an immune response to foods, infection, healing, and more.

Microbiome: All the microorganisms that reside in your body, including your digestive system. Research has also discovered that other tissues have a microbiome, such as the skin.

Migrating motor complex: These are waves that propel food from the stomach through the intestines to support normal gut function.

Paleo: A style of eating that mimics eating patterns in the Paleolithic period or around 10,000 years ago.

Phospholipids: are substances that help with cellular communication, help support cell membranes, and help protect our body from toxins.

Postbiotics: Compounds made by the microbiome or from probiotics; they can also be given as supplements.

Proton pump inhibitors (PPIs): Prescription medications that block the actions of enzymes in the stomach and reduce the amount of acid made there.

RDI (Reference Daily Intake) is a system of guidelines developed by the Food and Nutrition Board of the National Academies of Sciences Engineering, and Medicine. These are not geared towards making individuals healthy but based on average requirements based on antiquated research at times.

Short gut syndrome: A condition usually due to the removal of intestines during surgery. The body is then unable to absorb enough nutrients to thrive.

Short-chain fatty acids: A type of fat with fewer than six carbon atoms often made from the fermentation of fibers but also made by probiotics in the gut.

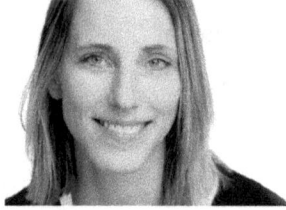

About the Author

Heidi Moretti, MS, RD, is a registered dietitian at Fresenius Medical Care and owns The Healthy RD LLC, a blog and resource for people looking for natural and scientifically proven remedies for health issues. She received post-graduate school training through the Institute for Functional Medicine and is constantly using the National Library of Medicine to uncover natural medicines research. She is the author of *The Whole Body Guide to Gut Health* and *The Elimination Diet Journal.* She has published numerous clinical research studies as the principal investigator for these studies, including:

"Vitamin D3 repletion versus placebo as adjunctive treatment of heart failure patient quality of life and hormonal indices: a randomized, double-blind, placebo-controlled trial."

"Biotin Deficiency as a target for treating restless legs syndrome in chronic dialysis patients."

"Effects of protein supplementation in chronic hemodialysis and peritoneal dialysis patients."

"Prevalence of low albumin, suboptimal energy, and muscle stores in Asian dialysis patients."

Additionally, she worked for over twenty years at Providence Saint Patrick Hospital in Missoula, where she honed her clinical skills and continued to find ways to add functional medicine into a conventional world.

You can connect with me on:

🌐 https://thehealthyrd.com

🐦 https://twitter.com/HeidiHmoretti

Subscribe to my newsletter:

✉ https://heidi-3842f.subscribemenow.com

Also by Heidi Moretti, MS, RD

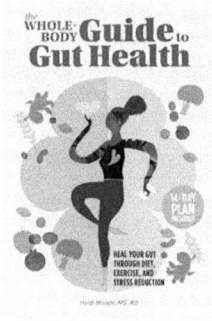

The Whole Body Guide to Gut Health

Your gut encompasses your digestive organs and all their resident microbes—and its health affects all the other systems in your body. Experience the physical and mental benefits of a healthy gut biome with this research-based guide. Find out how to care for your body, alleviate digestive distress, and soothe a wide variety of ailments, from heartburn and irritable bowel syndrome to depression and anxiety.

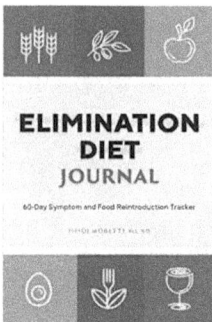

Elimination Diet Journal: 60-Day Symptom and Food Reintroduction Tracker

Your diet directly contributes to your health and sense of well-being, but some foods can cause inflammation, digestion issues, and aggravate autoimmune disorders. This journal will walk you through the elimination diet, giving you the tools and guidance to determine which foods are harming you and identify those that may help heal your gut.

Index

i

www.ingramcontent.com/pod-product-compliance
Lightning Source LLC
Chambersburg PA
CBHW070059030426
42335CB00016B/1948